Practical Guide to Female Pelvic Medicine

Dedication

From early in my career, there was one person whose words echo in my mind: 'Write the paper!', 'Give the talk!'. Although I cursed the words at the time, the importance of doing research and teaching our fellow physicians and colleagues has since become increasingly clear. Jamie MacGregor, MD, became not only my friend, but also my academic role model. I am forever grateful for his guidance, friendship and encouragement.

G Willy Davila

This book would not be possible without the loving support of my family. To my wife, Magda, who, after 25 years of love and support, is still my strength, my trusted advisor and my inspiration. To my son, Ashraf, and my daughter, Neehal, with a heart full of love.

Gamal Ghoniem

Practical Guide to Female Pelvic Medicine

Edited by

Gamal Ghoniem MD FACS
Head, Section of Voiding Dysfunction
Female Urology and Reconstruction
Cleveland Clinic Florida
Weston, FL
USA

G Willy Davila MD
Head, Section of Urogynecology and Reconstructive Pelvic Surgery
Department of Gynecology
Cleveland Clinic Florida
Weston, FL
USA

informa
healthcare

Informa Healthcare USA, Inc.
52 Vanderbilt Avenue
New York, NY 10017

© 2010 by Informa Healthcare USA, Inc. (original copyright 2006 by the Taylor & Fracis Group)
Informa Healthcare is an Informa business

No claim to original U.S. Government works

10 9 8 7 6 5 4 3 2 1

International Standard Book Number-10: 1-8418-4398-8 (Hardcover)
International Standard Book Number-13: 978-1-8418-4398-8 (Hardcover)

Visit the Informa Web site at
www.informa.com

and the Informa Healthcare Web site at
www.informahealthcare.com

Contents

Contributors

Chahin Achtari MD
Unité d'Urodynamique
Maternité CHUV
1011 Lausanne
Switzerland

Alfred E Bent MD
Department of Obstetrics and Gynecology
Dalhousie University
Halifax, NS
Canada

Daniel Biller MD
Section of Urogynecology and Reconstructive Surgery
Department of Gynecology
Cleveland Clinic Florida
Weston, FL
USA

Linda Cardozo MD FRCOG
Professor of Urogynaecology
King's College Hospital
London
UK

G Willy Davila MD
Head, Section of Urogynecology and Reconstructive Pelvic Surgery
Department of Gynecology
Cleveland Clinic Florida
Weston, FL
USA

Peter L Dwyer MD
Urogynaecology Department
Mercy Hospital for Women
Victoria
Australia

Gamal Ghoniem MD FACS
Head, Section of Voiding Dysfunction
Female Urology and Reconstruction
Clinical Professor of Surgery/Urology – NSU, OSU, and USF
Cleveland Clinic Florida
Weston, FL
USA

Lawrence S Hakim MD FACS
Head, Section of Sexual Medicine, Infertility and Prosthetics
Cleveland Clinic Florida
Weston, FL
USA

Melissa E Huggins MD
Clinical Instructor
University of California
Irvine College of Medicine
Irvine, CA
USA

Jose Marcio N Jorge MD
Associate Professor
Department of Coloproctology
University of São Paulo
Brazil

Dharmesh S Kapoor MD
Subspecialist trainee in Urogynecology
Derriford Hospital
Plymouth
UK

Erin E Katz MD
Clincal Fellow
Department of Urology
Cleveland Clinic Florida
Weston, FL
USA

Jonathan D Kaye MD
Long Island Jewish Medical Center
New Hyde Park, NY
USA

Usama Khater MD
Research Fellow
Department of Urology
Cleveland Clinic Florida
Weston, FL
USA

Neeraj Kohli MD MBA
Chief Director
Division of Urogynecology
Brigham and Women's Hospital
Harvard Medical School
Boston, MA
USA

Robert M Moldwin MD
Director, Interstitial Cystitis Center
Long Island Jewish Medical Center
New Hyde Park, NY
USA

Donald R Ostergard MD FACOG
Professor of Obstetrics and Gynecology
Department of Obstetrics and Gynecology
University of California
Irvine College of Medicine
Irvine, CA
and
Director, Division of Urogynecology
Department of Obstetrics and Gynecology
Associate Medical Director for Gynecology
Long Beach Memorial Women's Hospital
Long Beach, CA
USA

Johann Pfeifer MD
Associate Professor of Surgery
Department of General Surgery
Medical University of Graz
Graz
Austria

Sujatha Rajan MD
Division of Urogynecology
Brigham and Women's Hospital
Harvard Medical School
Boston, MA
USA

Dudley Robinson MD MRCOG
Consultant Obstetrician and Urogynaecologist
Department of Urogynaecology
Kings College Hospital
London
UK

Yishai Ron MD
Director, Gastrointestinal Motility Unit
E Wolfson Medical Center
Holon
and
Sackler School of Medicine
Tel Aviv University
Tel Aviv
Israel

Nirit Rosenblum MD
Assistant Professor of Urology
Department of Urology
New York University School of Medicine
New York, NY
USA

Hagit Tulchinsky MD
Colon and Rectal Surgery
Proctology Unit
Division of Surgery B
Tel Aviv-Sourasky Medical Center
Tel Aviv
Israel

Brian A VanderBrink MD
Long Island Jewish Medical Center
New Hyde Park, NY
USA

Eric Weiss MD
Department of Colorectal Surgery
Cleveland Clinic Florida
Weston, FL
USA

Samir Yebara MD
Department of Colorectal Surgery
Cleveland Clinic Florida
Weston, FL
USA

Oded Zmora MD
Colon and Rectal Surgery
Department of Surgery and Transplantation
Sheba Medical Center
Tel Hashomer
Israel

Foreword

One might ask, why another book on pelvic floor disorders, and what does this text have to offer that others might not? In my opinion, this is an extremely well-organized and orchestrated text that concentrates more so on practical matters, as opposed to theory, than other texts in the field, and is consequently geared towards residents, fellows and practitioners. The editors are experienced and expert clinicians and educators, and have had ample experience in other venues in separating the wheat from the chaff. The chapters are all written by very experienced international teachers, the information is up-to-date, and an obvious effort has been made to distill practical information into summaries, figures and tables. Each chapter contains essential information for understanding and implementing the basis and practicalities of good practice, the value and interpretation of various investigations, and, where applicable, the specifics of choosing and implementing proper therapy. A Venn diagram describing the text would include female urology, urogynecology and colorectal considerations. My compliments to the editors for their orchestration of a text that will prove to be very useful and heavily utilized.

Alan J Wein MD

Preface

Female pelvic floor disorders have become an area of greater investigation as the segment of the aging population increases. Most of these disorders are not life threatening, and thus were slow to be studied or practiced. Moreover, different specialists treated disorders as separate anatomical entities, often not addressing neighboring compartments and their interaction. This longitudinal concept of separate systems – urological, gynecological and colorectal – is now pointless in favor of a more transverse concept of the female pelvic organs as a functional unit. With the wealth of programs dedicated to advanced training in female pelvic medicine, surgeons will provide comprehensive and better care of our patients with emphasis on quality of life. However, diseases of the female pelvic floor cause significant social, psychological and economic burdens and may generate major distress and embarrassment to the patients. The demand for better quality of life, along with the growing segment of patients suffering from pelvic floor disorders has pushed the interest to the forefront. Currently, it is very rapidly changing with improvement in understanding, diagnosing and treating these disorders. This practical text will present to the reader a current state of the art with respect to evaluation and management.

The busy physician who is interested and practicing in this field needs a current and practical reference for his or her practice, and this work was created with this in mind. The contributing authors are made up of urologists, urogynecologists, gynecologists and colorectal surgeons, and are well-known international physicians with extensive experience in diagnosing and treating diseases and disorders of the pelvic floor as an integral unit.

As a multiauthor text, this book rapidly came to fruition. Our fellows have been a source of continuous stimulation, questions and fresh ideas, all of which have materialized in this work. The editors wish to thank the authors for their contributions and timely submission of their work.

Gamal Ghoniem
G Willy Davila

Acknowledgments

I am grateful to many individuals, colleagues and fellows who inspired me to edit such a book. Many thanks and sincere gratitude to our academic coordinator, Kristin Dunn, for hours of arduous and dedicated work. Thanks also to Alan Burgess, Senior Publisher at Taylor & Francis Medical Books, and Oliver Walter, Development Editor, for their continuous encouragement, advice and expertise.

Gamal Ghoniem

Color plates

The following figures are color versions of selected figures from the main body of the text.

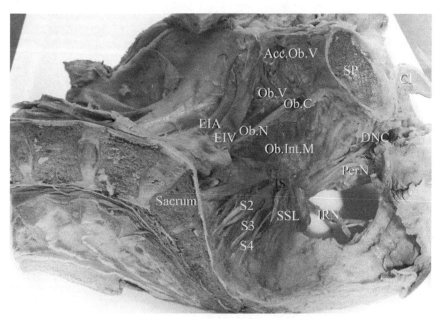

Figure 1.5 Left hemipelvis, medial view. The levator ani muscle has been removed and Alcock's canal has been opened to demonstrate the branches of the pudendal nerve.
IS = ischial spine, SSL = sacrospinous ligament, IRN = inferior rectal nerve, PerN = perineal nerve, DNC = dorsal nerve of clitoris, CI = clitoris, SP = symphysis pubis, Ob.N = obturator nerve, Ob.C = obturator canal, Ob.Int.M = obturator internus muscle, Ob.V = obturator vein, Acc.Ob.V = accessory obturator vein, EIV = external iliac vein, EIA = external iliac artery, S2–S4 = sacral roots.

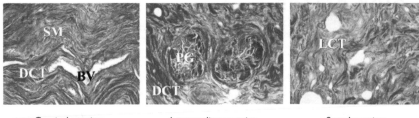

Cervical portion   Intermediate portion   Sacral portion

Figure 1.8 Microscopic view (40×) of the different portions of uterosacral ligaments. DCT = dense connective tissue made of collagen and elastin fibers. SM = smooth muscle fibers and fibroblasts, PG = parasympathetic ganglion, LCT = loose connective tissue, BV = blood vessel.

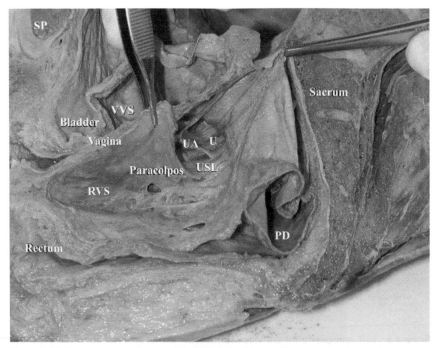

Figure 1.10 Retroperitoneal view of vaginal vault support. The upper vagina and cervix are attached to the pelvic sidewall by the paracolpos and lateral and uterosacral ligaments complex (USL). Also note the position of the ureter (U) running anteriorly to the USL and crossing under the uterine artery (UA). VVS = vesicovaginal space, RVS = rectovaginal space, PD = pouch of Douglas.

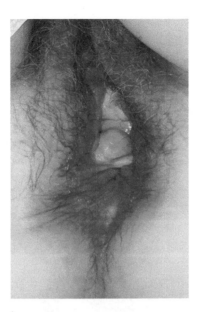

Figure 3.1 Incontinent patient after birth trauma. Note: the perineum is lost.

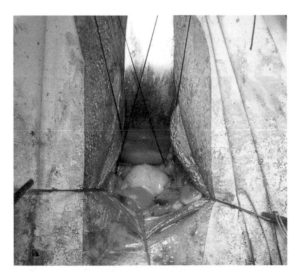

Figure 4.3 A McCall culdoplasty incorporates both uterosacral ligaments, intervening posterior cul-de-sac peritoneum, and full thickness of the apical vaginal wall.

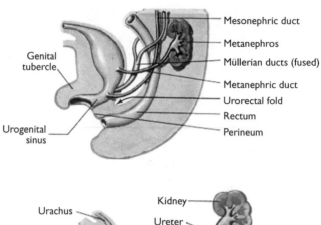

Mesonephric duct

Metanephros

Müllerian ducts (fused)

Metanephric duct

Urorectal fold

Rectum

Perineum

Genital
tubercle

Urogenital
sinus

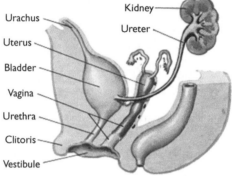

Kidney

Urachus

Ureter

Uterus

Bladder

Vagina

Urethra

Clitoris

Vestibule

Figure 5.1 Embryologic origin of the female genital and lower urinary tract.

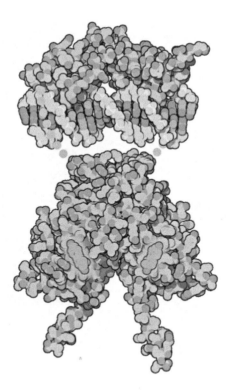

Figure 5.3 Estrogen receptor from the Molecule of the Month series by David S. Goodsell of The Scripps Research Institute http://www.rcsb.org/pdb/molecules/pdb45_1.html.

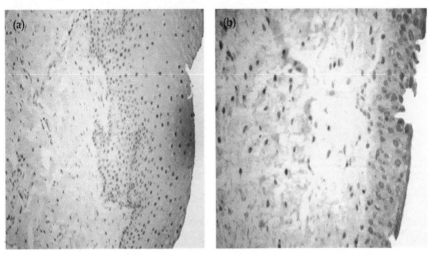

Figure 5.4 Estrogen receptors (stained dark blue) are present in the subepithelium of the vagina (a), although they have much lower expression in the bladder (b).

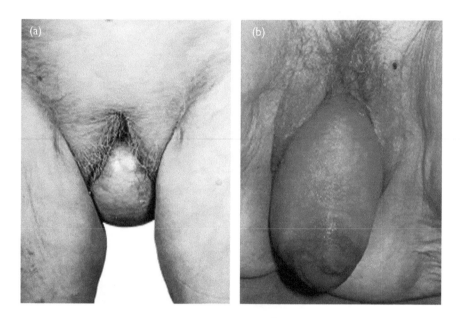

Figure 5.6 Vaginal vault prolapse (a) and third-degree uterine prolapse (b) in postmenopausal women complaining of urogenital atrophy.

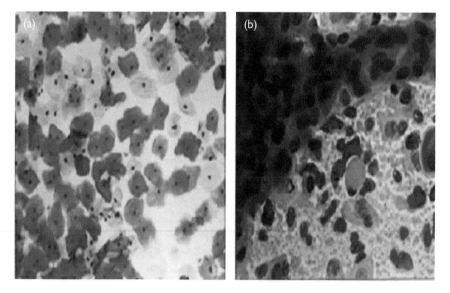

Figure 5.7 Vaginal cytology in a healthy premenopausal woman (a) and following the menopause in a woman with symptomatic vaginal atrophy (b).

(a) 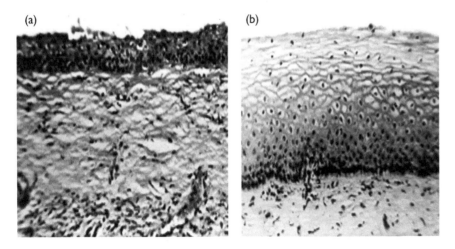 (b)

Figure 5.10 Topical vaginal estrogen replacement increases the number of intermediate and superficial cells in the vaginal mucosa: (a) prior to treatment and (b) following treatment.

(a) 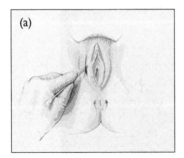 (b)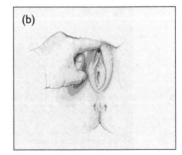

Figure 6.2 (a) Bulbocavernosus and (b) clitoral sacral reflexes. Lightly tapping the clitoris or brushing the labia majora should produce a reflex contraction of the external anal sphincter muscle. Reproduced with permission from Culligan PJ, Heit M. Urinary incontinence in women: evaluation and management. Am Fam Physician 2000;62(11): 2433–44.

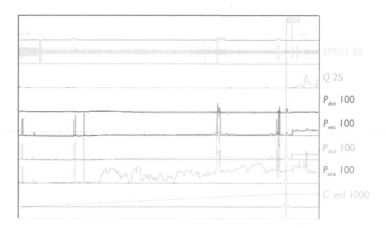

Figure 8.4 Multichannel cystometry showing a normal cystometrogram.

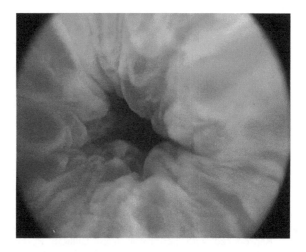

Figure 9.3 Normal urethral mucosa.

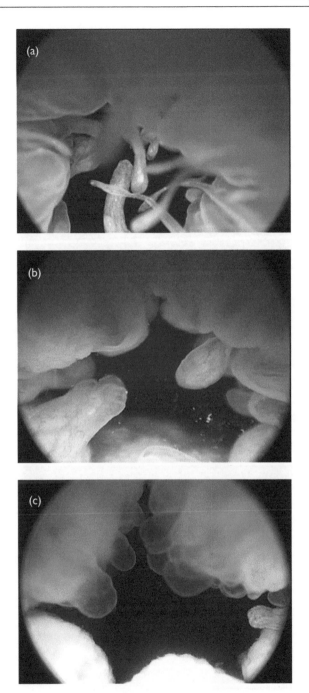

Figure 9.4 (a) Fronds, (b) polyps, and (c) cysts at the bladder neck.

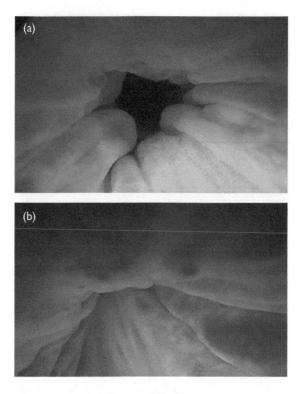

Figure 9.5 Maneuvers at bladder neck: (a) bladder neck open and (b) bladder neck closed.

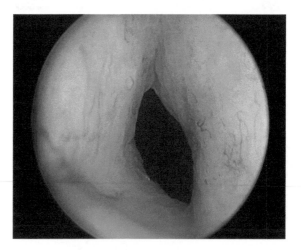

Figure 9.6 Scarred bladder neck.

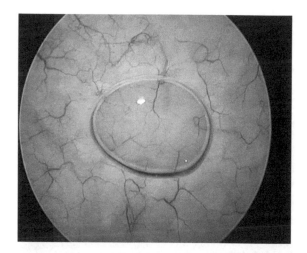

Figure 9.7 Normal bladder wall.

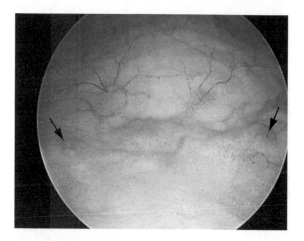

Figure 9.8 Bladder trigone (arrows mark uriteral orifices).

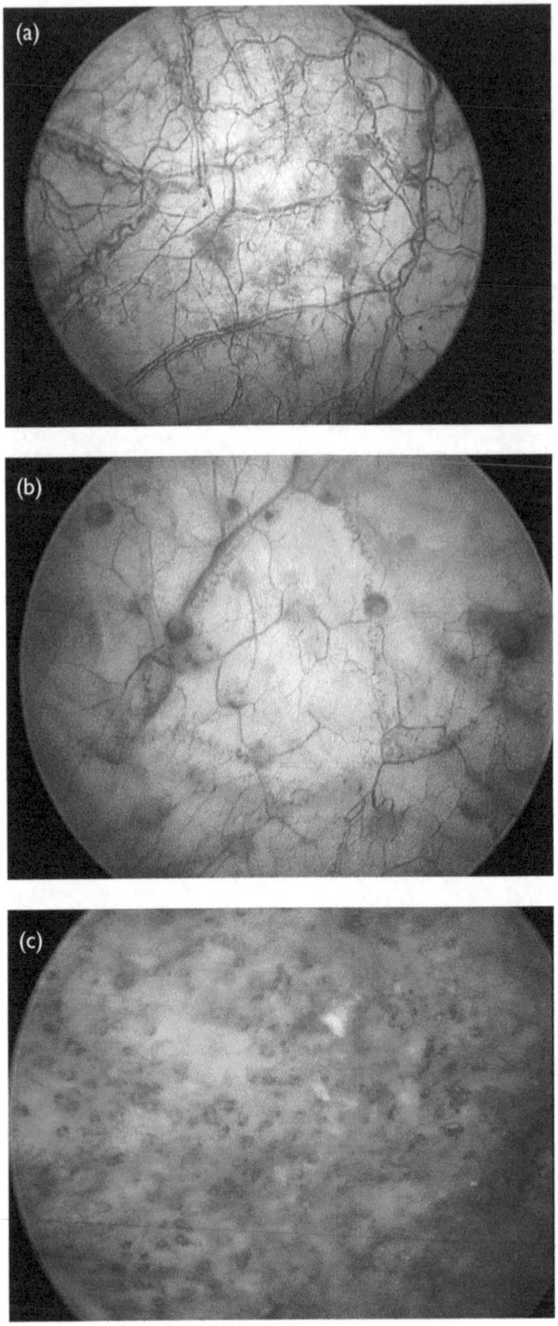

Figure 9.9 Abnormal mucosal surface of bladder: (a) spots of inflammation, (b) inflamed bladder wall, and (c) extensive inflammation of bladder wall.

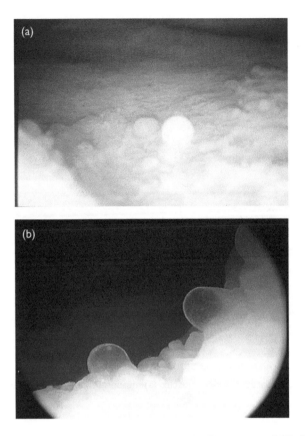

Figure 9.10 Cystitis cystica at trigone: (a) opaque and yellow cysts and (b) clear cysts.

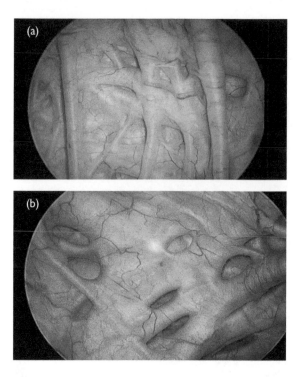

Figure 9.11 Trabeculated bladder muscle: (a) moderately severe and (b) severe with cellules.

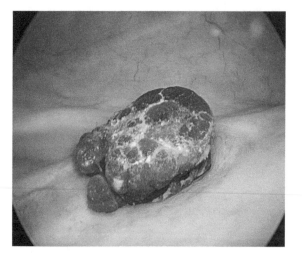

Figure 9.12 Bladder stone.

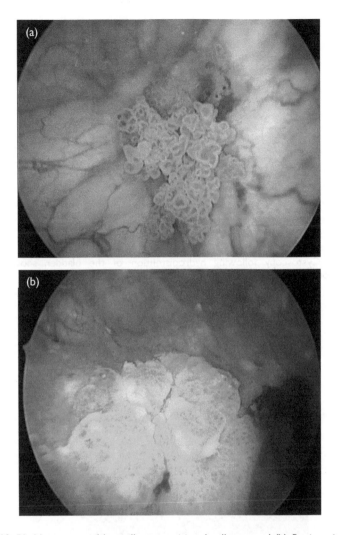

Figure 9.13 Bladder tumors: (a) papillary transitional cell type and (b) flat invasive type.

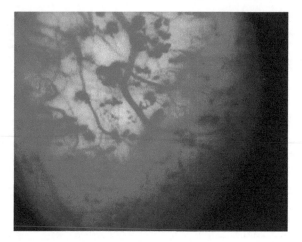

Figure 18.1 Cystoscopy following hydrodistention of the bladder, showing diffuse glomerulation.

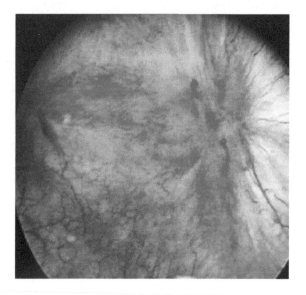

Figure 18.2 Hunner's ulcer.

Chapter 1

Pelvic floor anatomy

Chahin Achtari and Peter L Dwyer

Introduction

The aim of this chapter is to present an overview of the normal anatomy of the pelvis. This will provide the clinician with a better understanding of the function and support of pelvic organs and their relevance to modern urogynecologic practice.

Bony pelvis and ligaments

The intra-abdominal cavity extends from the diaphragm cranially to the pelvic floor caudally. When humans adopted the standing position, the gravitational effect of intra-abdominal pressure was transferred from the abdominal (as in quadrupeds) to the pelvic floor musculofascial complex. Muscles that quadrupeds contract voluntarily to move their tail have progressively evolved into supportive structures that require continual involuntary tonic contraction, but also need to provide rapid voluntary contraction for continence mechanisms to bladder and bowel.

The bony pelvis is composed by two coxal bones, the sacrum and the coccyx. Each coxal bone is composed by the fusion of the pubis, ischium, and ilium (Figure 1.1). Anteriorly, coxal bones are tightly attached to each other at the symphysis pubis and posteriorly to the sacrum at the sacroiliac junction. Pubic bones have two branches each: the inferior pubic rami fused with the ischium and the superior pubic rami fused with the ilium. The area circumscribed by the pubic rami and the ischium is the obturator foramen, which has a strong connective tissue membrane (the obturator membrane), with the obturator neurovascular bundle on its superior-lateral aspect (the obturator canal).

Two strong ligaments arise from the lateral margins of the sacrum: the sacrotuberous ligament, attaching to the ischial tuberosity; and the sacrospinous ligament, which attaches to the ischial spine (Figure 1.2). The iliopectineal ligament runs along the superior margin of the internal surface of the superior pubic rami. It has no supportive role, but is used as

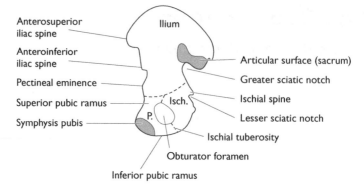

Figure 1.1 Right coxal bone, medial view. P = pubic bone, Isch = ischial bone. Note that in the standing position, the anterosuperior iliac spine and the anterior margin of the pubic bone lie in the same vertical plane.

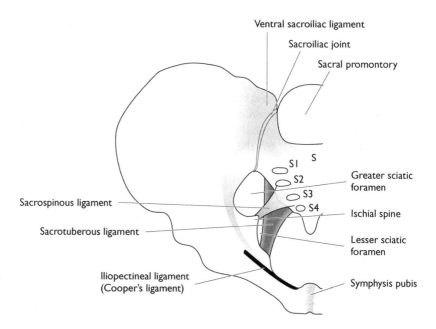

Figure 1.2 Right hemipelvis and ligaments, anterior superior view. S = sacrum, S1–4 = sacral foramina.

an anchoring structure in some anti-incontinence procedures (e.g. Burch colposuspension).

The ischial spine is an important landmark and is easily palpable through the vagina or rectum. It plays a central role in pelvic floor support as an anchoring structure for several important ligaments. The *sacrospinous liga-*

ment has an important role in pelvic reconstructive surgery for it can be used as an anchoring structure during vaginal vault suspension (sacrospinous vaginal vault suspension). The sacrospinous ligament separates the greater from the lesser sciatic foramen. The *arcus tendineus levator ani* (ATLA) is the lateral tendinous attachment of the levator ani muscle and extends anteriorly from the internal aspect of pubic bone, running along the pelvic sidewall to attach posteriorly to the ischial spine. Finally, the endopelvic fascia that supports pelvic organs is attached to the *arcus tendineus fascia pelvis* (ATFP), a band of dense connective tissue running from the back of the pubic symphysis to the ischial spine (Figure 1.3).

Pelvic floor muscles and nerve supply

Pelvic floor muscles (or levator ani muscle) are divided into two main portions: the pubovisceralis medially; the iliococcygeus and coccygeus laterally and posteriorly. These are paired structures that are fused together in the midline. Puborectalis muscle is the bulkiest and most medial aspect of the pubovisceralis muscle. It arises from the back of the pubic bone and runs almost horizontally to wrap like a sling around the back of the anorectal junction, elevating the rectum and other pelvic organs cranially and anteriorly. Its medial border forms the urogenital hiatus through which urethra, vagina,

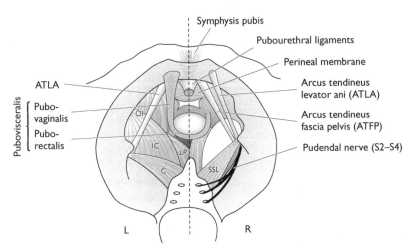

Figure 1.3 Pelvic floor muscles and ligamentous support, superior view. On the right side, pelvic floor muscles have been removed to demonstrate important ligaments inserting on the ischial spine (SSL = sacrospinous ligament, ATLA, and ATFP). The pudendal nerve exits the pelvic cavity through the greater sciatic foramen, turns around the ischial spine, and re-enters the pelvic cavity through the lesser sciatic foramen. On the left side, pubovisceralis gives fibers to the vagina and rectum. PC = pubococcygeus forming posteriorly with the iliococcygeus (IC) the levator plate (LP). OI = obturator internus muscle.

and anal canal pass. It gives muscular fibers to these structures and is therefore divided into specific portions called pubovaginalis and puborectalis (Figure 1.3).

Pubococcygeus is the lateral part of pubovisceralis muscle. It arises from the back of the pubic bone and anterior part of the ATLA. Pubococcygeus connects pubis with coccyx and is fused with its counterpart along the median raphe, which runs from the back of the rectum to the coccyx. Laterally and posteriorly lies the iliococcygeus muscle, which is a thinner layer of muscle arising from the ATLA and is also fused with its counterpart along the median raphe and attached posteriorly to the coccyx. Together with the pubococcygeus, they provide a shelf called the 'levator plate' on which pelvic organs rest. The coccygeus muscle forms the posterior part of the pelvic diaphragm. It runs from the ischial spine to the coccyx and lower sacrum. Its superior and posterior aspect is made of dense connective tissue forming the sacrospinous ligament (Figure 1.3).

The pelvic diaphragm refers to the levator ani and coccygeus muscles with their superior and inferior fasciae. The perineal membrane (urogenital diaphragm) refers to a triangular layer of dense connective tissue lying inferiorly to the pelvic diaphragm in the anterior pelvic triangle. It attaches distal urethra, vagina, and perineal body to the inferior pubic rami. Superficial to the perineal membrane are the ischiocavernosus, the bulbocavernosus, and the superficial transverse muscles completing the inferior aspect of urogenital diaphragm (Figure 1.4). Posteriorly, there is no equivalent to the perineal membrane. The external anal sphincter lies in this plane attached anteriorly to the superficial transverse perinei and bulbocavernosus, forming the perineal body, and posteriorly to the coccyx.

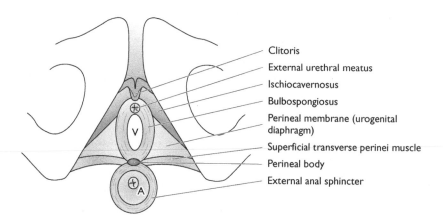

Clitoris
External urethral meatus
Ischiocavernosus
Bulbospongiosus
Perineal membrane (urogenital diaphragm)
Superficial transverse perinei muscle
Perineal body
External anal sphincter

Figure 1.4 Superficial perineal muscles. V = vagina, A = anus.

The pudendal nerve provides the pelvic floor somatic innervation, arising from the sacral roots S2–S4. The pudendal nerve exits the pelvic cavity through the greater sciatic foramen, passes behind the ischial spine and sacrospinous ligament and re-enters the pelvic space through the lesser sciatic foramen. It then enters into the pudendal (Alcock's) canal formed by the duplication of obturator internus membrane along the inferior pubic ramus (Figure 1.5). The pudendal nerve gives three branches:

- The first branch is the inferior rectal nerve that arises at the beginning of the pudendal canal and penetrates the ischiorectal fossa. It gives motor branches to the lower rectum and the external anal sphincter, and sensory branches to the skin anterior and lateral to the anus.
- The second branch of the pudendal nerve, the perineal nerve, arises from the middle of the pudendal canal and gives a sensory perineal branch and a motor branch for the external urethral sphincter and perineal muscles.

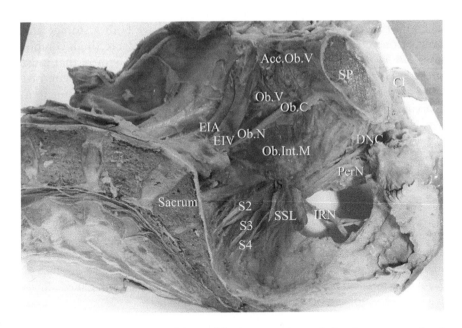

Figure 1.5 Left hemipelvis, medial view. The levator ani muscle has been removed and Alcock's canal has been opened to demonstrate the branches of the pudendal nerve. IS = ischial spine, SSL = sacrospinous ligament, IRN = inferior rectal nerve, PerN = perineal nerve, DNC = dorsal nerve of clitoris, Cl = clitoris, SP = symphysis pubis, Ob.N = obturator nerve, Ob.C = obturator canal, Ob.Int.M = obturator internus muscle, Ob.V = obturator vein, Acc.Ob.V = accessory obturator vein, EIV = external iliac vein, EIA = external iliac artery, S2–S4 = sacral roots. (See also color image on p. xvii)

- The terminal branch of the pudendal nerve is the dorsal nerve of the clitoris that crosses the infrapubic canal and supplies sensory innervation to the clitoral area.

Levator ani muscle is innervated on its internal surface by branches directly derived from S3 to S4 forming the levator ani nerve, without contribution from the pudendal nerve.[1,2]

The autonomic nerve supply of the pelvic organs plays an important role in their sphincter mechanism. The inferior hypogastric plexus is composed of a confluence of nerves from the superior hypogastric plexus (parasympathetic), the pelvic sympathetic plexus (a direct continuation from the lumbar trunk), and the pelvic splanchnic nerves (parasympathetic, nervi erigentes) arising directly from the second, third, and fourth sacral foramina. This nerve plexus runs along the lateral sides of the rectum, vagina, and bladder and provides autonomic innervation to these organs and to their sphincters.

Pelvic organs

The lower urinary tract and the rectoanal canal have both a storage and evacuation role. They distend without increase of pressure (high compliance) whilst maintaining continence by a sphincter mechanism that must provide both long-term tonic and rapid phasic contraction. In contrast during evacuation, the organs must be able to contract with sphincteric relaxing in a coordinated fashion.

Ureters

Ureters are muscular tubes conveying urine from the kidneys to the bladder. Their abdominal course is retroperitoneal anteromedial to the psoas muscle. They cross under the ovarian vessels at variable levels between the aortic and iliac bifurcation and then run parallel to them. The ureters enter the pelvic cavity by crossing over the external iliac vessels, and run along the pelvic sidewall in the pararectal space, anterior to the hypogastric artery and the uterosacral ligaments. They cross under the uterine artery along a distance of 2.5 cm about 2 cm lateral to the vaginal fornices, finally inclining medially to reach the base of the bladder in front of the vagina.

Bladder

The bladder is a preperitoneal organ composed of smooth muscle (the detrusor muscle), covered on its dome by a serosal layer and lined by a submucosa and transitional cell epithelium. The detrusor muscle is composed of three separate bundles of smooth muscle arranged in an internal and external longitudinal and an intermediate circular layer. The bladder wall is traversed by the two ureters at its posterolateral angles. Ureters run obliquely within the bladder wall at a distance of 1.5–2 cm and open into the bladder cavity at the ureteric orifices. These ureteric orifices superiorly and the internal urethral meatus inferiorly mark the limits of the trigone at the base of the bladder. The bladder base rests posteriorly on the vagina. The dome of the bladder is covered by peritoneum (Figure 1.6), which extends posteriorly as far as the isthmus of the uterus, onto which it is reflected to form the uterovesical pouch. Anteriorly, the bladder lies in the retropubic space, which is filled with adipose and loose areolar tissue.

Urethra

The urethra is a fibromuscular tube measuring 3–4 cm that extends from the vesical neck to the external urethral meatus. Its mucosa is a transitional cell urothelium in its upper third and a nonkeratinizing squamous epithelium in its distal two-thirds. Urinary continence is maintained by urethral pressure that exceeds intravesical pressure. The sphincter is composed of an internal smooth and an external striated muscle distributed in different proportions along its course. Smooth muscle is present along the upper two-thirds of the urethral length. The striated urethral sphincter is circular on the upper two-thirds and includes the compressor urethrae and the urethrovaginal sphincter distally (Figures 1.7a, 1.7b), just above the urogenital diaphragm.[3] A well-developed layer of submucosal vessels also participates in the continence mechanism. Arteriovenous anastomoses

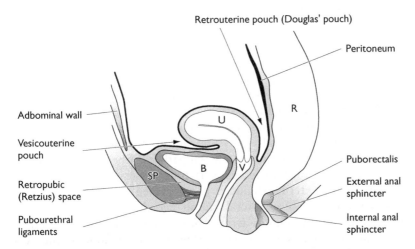

Figure 1.6 Pelvic organs and peritoneal lining. SP = symphysis pubis, B = bladder, U = uterus, R = rectum, V = vagina.

(a)

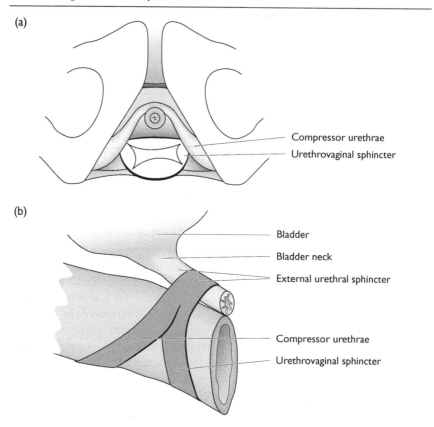

Compressor urethrae
Urethrovaginal sphincter

(b)

Bladder
Bladder neck
External urethral sphincter

Compressor urethrae
Urethrovaginal sphincter

Figure 1.7 (a) Deep perineal muscles (after Oelrich[3]), interior view. (b) External urethral sphincter and deep perineal muscles, lateral view.

allow inflation of venules, which provide watertight mucosal coaptation and increase the closure pressure of the urethra. These vessels, as well as urethral and trigonal mucosa, have estrogen and progesterone receptors.[4]

The urethral sphincter muscles are under complex neurologic control, involving the pudendal (afferent) and autonomic nerves.[5] The smooth internal sphincter is innervated by sympathetic fibers arising from the ventral lumbar region that increase its tone via α_1-noradrenergic receptors. The striated external sphincter is innervated by somatic nerves arising from the caudal lumbosacral region via cholinergic receptors. The afferent limb of this lumbosacral reflex is mediated by the pudendal nerve, which stimulates the efferent pathway during bladder filling. At the same time, this lumbosacral reflex (the guarding reflex) is modulated by reflex pontine and voluntary central control.

The urethra is supported posteriorly by the vaginal wall and is fused with it at its terminal third. Anteriorly, the urethra is suspended to the pubic bone by the pubourethral ligaments[6] and is attached laterally to the pubovisceralis muscle through a layer of endopelvic fascia. These muscular and ligamentous supports prevent urethral opening during rises of intra-abdominal pressure.[7]

Genital tract

The vagina, which is essentially a muscular tubular organ lined by a non-keratinizing squamous epithelium, occupies a central position in the female pelvis. The bladder and urethra are positioned anteriorly to the vagina, the rectum and anal canal posteriorly, and the cervix cranially.

The uterus is divided into a body (corpus) and a cervix. The body is pear-shaped and narrows from its fundus at the level of the internal cervical os. On either side of the fundus, uterine (Fallopian) tubes carry ova from the ovaries to the uterine cavity through the ostia. The round ligaments are attached to the fundus anteriorly and the tubes and the utero-ovarian ligaments posteriorly. The uterus is covered by peritoneum (Figure 1.7) that extends laterally over the round ligament to form the broad ligaments, stretching from the sides of the uterus to the lateral pelvic sidewall.

The cervix is approximately 2.5 cm long. The vagina inserts onto the distal part of the cervix dividing it into an intravaginal and a supravaginal portion.

Rectum

The terminal digestive tract is formed by the rectum and the anal canal. The rectum functions as a reservoir and the anal canal maintains continence. The transition between rectum and anal canal is at the level of the pelvic diaphragm. Peritoneum covers the upper two-thirds of the rectum anteriorly and is reflected onto the upper posterior vaginal wall, forming the rectovaginal pouch of Douglas. The rectal mucosa consists of columnar and mucus-producing cells that also line the upper anal canal down to the dentate line. Under this line the anal epithelium is a nonkeratinized stratified squamous epithelium of the perianal epidermis.

Anal canal

The anal canal is approximately 4 cm long, and in its wall there is an internal anal sphincter of smooth muscle, which is a continuation of the circular rectal muscularis. The puborectalis muscle is fused with the deep or upper part of the external anal sphincter. The superficial portion of the external anal sphincter is circular and is wrapped around the terminal portion of the internal anal sphincter. The terminal part of the external anal sphincter is a subcutaneous muscle, which is situated below the internal anal sphincter. In the intersphincteric space between the internal and external anal sphincter descends an extension of the longitudinal rectal muscularis, forming the conjoined longitudinal muscle.

The external anal sphincter is innervated by the inferior rectal nerve, a branch of the pudendal nerve. The internal anal sphincter has a sympathetic (motor) and parasympathetic (inhibitory) innervation. Distention of the rectum provokes relaxation of the internal anal sphincter (rectoanal inhibitory reflex) and contraction of the external anal sphincter (rectoanal contractile reflex).

Anal continence mainly relies upon anatomic and functional integrity of the anal sphincter mechanism. The internal anal sphincter provides about 80% of resting pressure. The external anal sphincter is composed of slow-twitch and fast-twitch fibers and contributes to about 20% of resting tone, although its role is to generate rapid voluntary contraction.[8]

The endopelvic fascia and pelvic floor support

The levator ani muscles are the primary pelvic organ supports and provide a muscular plate upon which they can rest. Levator ani is composed of slow-twitch, fatigue-resistant fibers that maintain constant tone and fast-twitch fibers that allow rapid contraction with sudden rises in intra-abdominal pressure. Loss of muscular support caused by either denervation or direct muscular damage will impose increased load on pelvic connective tissue and provoke a progressive sliding of pelvic organs through the urogenital hiatus. Pelvic organ prolapse is therefore closely related to the integrity of pelvic floor muscles and perivaginal connective tissue. Ligamentous support in the pelvis is provided by a retroperitoneal layer of connective tissue called endopelvic fascia (EPF), which represents the top layer of the pelvic floor. The term 'fascia' poorly defines the true composition of these local condensations of connective tissue that differs from other fasciae of the body. The composition of EPF varies with anatomic site but consists mainly of fibrocytes and fibroblasts, smooth muscle cells, collagen (mainly types I and III), elastin fibers, nerves, and blood vessels. EPF provides secondary support to the pelvic organs, by anchoring them to the pelvic sidewalls.

It is clinically useful to divide the upper vaginal and supravaginal cervix support into a posteromedial part, the uterosacral ligaments, and an anterolateral part, the cardinal ligaments. Uterosacral ligaments (USLs) have been extensively described by Campbell,[9] who divided them into a cervical, an intermediate, and a sacral portion (Figure 1.8). The cervical portion is attached to the posterolateral aspect of the cervix at the level of the internal os and to the lateral vaginal fornices. It is mainly composed of smooth muscle and connective tissue. It also contains sympathetic and parasympathetic nerve fibers. Its middle portion is made of a dense connective tissue

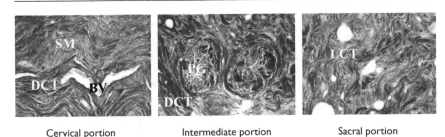

Cervical portion   Intermediate portion   Sacral portion

Figure 1.8 Microscopic view (40×) of the different portions of uterosacral ligaments. DCT = dense connective tissue made of collagen and elastin fibers. SM = smooth muscle fibers and fibroblasts, PG = parasympathetic ganglion, LCT = loose connective tissue, BV = blood vessel. (See also color image on p. xviii)

band, the 'stratum fibrosum' at its anterior margin and loose connective tissue posteriorly. Nerves and parasympathetic ganglia are also found at this level. The sacral portion is essentially made of loose connective tissue and fans out to insert on the presacral fascia. The direction of USLs is vertical and provides a suspension of the upper vagina and cervix. The cardinal ligaments (also called transverse cervical ligaments by Mackenrodt) are bands of dense connective tissue attaching the lateral margins of the cervix to the pelvic sidewalls. The uterine artery runs within this mass of tissue.

It is currently considered that these two ligaments represent different parts of the same complex of ligamentous tissue (Figure 1.9), suspending the upper third of the vagina and the cervix (level I). The paracolpium is the portion of EPF which attaches the vagina to the pelvic sidewall. The parametrium attaches the cervix laterally and posteriorly to the pelvic sidewall (Figure 1.10).[10] The paracolpium and parametrium prevent cervical and vaginal vault prolapse and are put under tension when traction is exerted on the cervix. The second third of the vagina (level II) is attached laterally to the ATFP through a sheet of EPF (Figure 1.8). This attachment stretches the vagina laterally and forms a continuous layer of support for the anterior pelvic compartment. The bladder is therefore supported posteriorly by a continuous layer composed by the vagina itself and its lateral insertions on the ATFP. Bladder anteriorly and rectum posteriorly are separated from the mid-vaginal wall by areolar tissue only. The rectovaginal septum is a layer of EPF attaching the posterior vaginal wall to the aponeurosis of levator ani muscle along a line extending along the pelvic sidewall from the perineal body to the middle of the ATFP.[11] The distal part of the vagina is fused (level III) with surrounding organs, anteriorly with the urethra, laterally to the pubovisceralis muscle and ischiopubic rami through the perineal membrane, and posteriorly with the perineal body.[12]

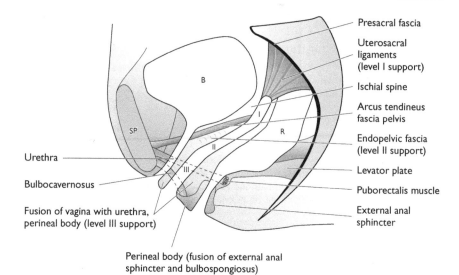

Figure 1.9 Vaginal support (after Delancey[10]). The vagina has three different levels of support. At level I, the vagina is suspended from the sacrum and pelvic sidewall by the paracolpos, the inferior extension of the uterosacral and laterocervical ligaments. At level II, the vagina lies in a more horizontal plane and is attached to the ATFP through a layer of endopelvic fascia. At level III, the vagina is again in a more vertical plane because of the action of the puborectalis muscle and is fused with surrounding organs and muscles.

Summary

- The pelvis is composed of the two coxal bones, the sacrum and the coccyx.
- The ischial spine is an easily palpable landmark on which several important ligaments insert: the arcus tendineus levator ani, the arcus tendineus fascia pelvis and the sacrospinous ligament.
- The levator ani muscles provide primary support to pelvic floor organs by elevating them anteriorly and providing a shelf (levator plate) on which they can rest posteriorly. The endopelvic fascia provides secondary support by attaching the pelvic organs to the pelvic sidewalls.
- The urethral and anal sphincters are both composed of an internal smooth muscle layer that provides resting tone and an external striated layer that can be contracted voluntarily.

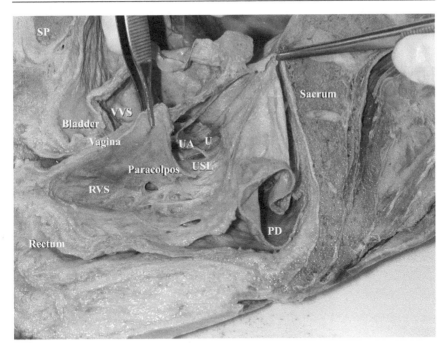

Figure 1.10 Retroperitoneal view of vaginal vault support. The upper vagina and cervix are attached to the pelvic sidewall by the paracolpos and lateral and uterosacral ligaments complex (USL). Also note the position of the ureter (U) running anteriorly to the USL and crossing under the uterine artery (UA). VVS = vesicovaginal space, RVS = rectovaginal space, PD = pouch of Douglas. (See also color image on p. xviii)

References

1. Barber MD, Bremer RE, Thor KB, et al. Innervation of the female levator ani muscles. Am J Obstet Gynecol 2002;187(1):64–71.
2. Matzel KE, Schmidt RA, Tanagho EA. Neuroanatomy of the striated muscular anal continence mechanism. Implications for the use of neurostimulation. Dis Colon Rectum 1990;33(8):666–73.
3. Oelrich TM. The striated urogenital sphincter muscle in the female. Anat Rec 1983;205(2):223–32.
4. Blakeman PJ, Hilton P, Bulmer JN. Oestrogen and progesterone receptor expression in the female lower urinary tract, with reference to oestrogen status. BJU Int 2000;86(1):32–8.
5. Fraser MO, Chancellor MB. Neural control of the urethra and development of pharmacotherapy for stress urinary incontinence. BJU Int 2003;91(8):743–8.
6. Zacharin RF. The anatomic supports of the female urethra. Obstet Gynecol 1968;32(6):754–9.
7. DeLancey JO. Structural support of the urethra as it relates to stress urinary incontinence: the hammock hypothesis. Am J Obstet Gynecol 1994;170(6): 1713–20.

8. Rao SS. Pathophysiology of adult fecal incontinence. Gastroenterology 2004;126(1 Suppl 1):S14–22.
9. Campbell RM. The anatomy and histology of the sacrouterine ligaments. Am J Obstet Gynecol 1950;59(1):1–12.
10. DeLancey JO. Anatomic aspects of vaginal eversion after hysterectomy. Am J Obstet Gynecol 1992;166(6 Pt 1):1717–24; discussion 1724–8.
11. Leffler KS, Thompson JR, Cundiff GW, et al. Attachment of the rectovaginal septum to the pelvic sidewall. Am J Obstet Gynecol 2001;185(1):41–3.
12. DeLancey JO. Structural anatomy of the posterior pelvic compartment as it relates to rectocele. Am J Obstet Gynecol 1999;180(4):815–23.

Chapter 2

Pathophysiology of urinary incontinence

Melissa E Huggins and Donald R Ostergard

Introduction

To understand the etiology of urinary incontinence in women, one must have a working knowledge of the interrelated roles of genitourinary neurophysiology, biomechanics, and anatomy in the intricate process of micturition.[1] Anatomic and neurologic pathology can occur during the life cycle of the female patient, with childbearing, hormonal changes, surgical intervention, and aging. The site of pathologic injury in this complex system determines the type of incontinence that will result. Types of incontinence and their definitions are shown in Table 2.1.

Physiology of micturition

Under normal circumstances, micturition is under voluntary control. The desire to void in a socially acceptable place is determined by the central nervous system. It provides input to the pontine micturition center located in the cerebellum. This center initiates the events that lead to micturition through efferent impulses to the lumbosacral spinal cord that exert both facilitatory and inhibitory signals to coordinate the somatic and autonomic nervous systems.

To facilitate urine storage, the somatic nervous system maintains closure of the proximal and mid-urethra, via the pudendal nerve.[2] The pudendal nerve innervates the rhabdosphincter, levator ani and fascia of the pelvic diaphragm.[3] The rhabdosphincter is considered the 'external' urethral sphincter, and is composed of a circumferential organization of striated muscle with attachments in the lateral vaginal wall.[4] This sphincter must voluntarily relax in order to allow bladder emptying. The levator ani muscle group exerts tonic pressure against the urethra to maintain continence.[4] In the presence of a stressful intra-abdominal force, contraction of the rhabdosphincter pulls the distal urethra (compressor urethra) towards the perineal body and rectum to further compress the urethra. At the same time the proximal urethra is elevated through its attachment to the arcus

Table 2.1 Incontinence types and definitions[9]

Stress urinary incontinence – the complaint of involuntary leakage on effort or exertion, or on sneezing or coughing

Urge urinary incontinence – the complaint of involuntary leakage accompanied by or immediately preceded by urgency

Mixed incontinence – the complaint of involuntary leakage associated with urgency and also with exertion, effort, sneezing, or coughing

Detrusor overactivity incontinence – incontinence due to an involuntary detrusor contraction is a urodynamic observation characterized by involuntary detrusor contractions during filling

Neurogenic detrusor overactivity – detrusor overactivity incontinence due to a relevant neurologic condition, which may be spontaneous or provoked

Idiopathic detrusor overactivity – detrusor overactivity incontinence without a defined cause

Urethral relaxation incontinence – leakage due to urethral relaxation in the presence of raised abdominal pressure or detrusor overactivity

Extraurethral incontinence – an observation of urine leakage through channels other than the urethra

Uncategorized incontinence – the observation of involuntary leakage that cannot be classified into one of the above categories, e.g. overflow incontinence from obstruction

---

tendineus fasciae pelvis.[5] In addition to the rhabdosphincter, the involuntary (smooth muscle) internal sphincter (bladder neck and proximal urethra) and the urethral submucosal vascular plexus contribute to maintain closure of the urethra.[6]

To initiate voiding, voluntary relaxation of the rhabdosphincter must occur. The parasympathetic system mediates inhibition of the resting tone of the smooth muscle at the bladder neck and along the urethra via the pelvic nerve, resulting in relaxation of an effective internal urethral sphincter. Parasympathetic fibers travel from S2 to S4 via the pelvic nerve (hypogastric nerve), to innervate the detrusor muscle. When stimulated, these fibers release acetylcholine, which binds to the M2 and M3 receptors, stimulating contraction of the smooth muscle fibers.[7] Of the 5 types of muscarinic receptors identified (M1–M5), the smooth muscle of the human bladder contains 80% M2 receptors. The remaining receptors are M3 type and are mainly responsible for detrusor muscle contraction.[8]

In contrast, the major role of the sympathetic nervous system is accommodating bladder filling by opposing the actions of the parasympathetic system through the β and α receptors. The α receptors are located at the bladder neck and along the urethra, while the β receptors are dispersed throughout the detrusor muscle. The sympathetic nerve roots originate in T11 through L2 and utilize the neurotransmitter norepinephrine. Sympathetic stimulation of the α-adrenergic receptors increases outlet resistance by stimulating the internal urethral sphincter to contract. Action on the β-adrenergic receptors cause bladder smooth muscle relaxation, inhibiting detrusor contractions. The sensation of bladder fullness is mediated through afferent nerves, which include myelinated Aδ fibers and unmyelinated C fibers, of the sympathetic and parasympathetic systems.[7]

Stress urinary incontinence (SUI) occurs when external forces placed on the bladder, such as with a cough or sneeze, exceed the closure pressure of the urethra. The mechanisms that maintain the urethral pressure are dependent on the intra-abdominal location of the urethra (Figure 2.1). Vaginal prolapse and urethral hypermobility can occur with the loss of supportive structures at the bladder neck and urethra. Intra-abdominal pressures with coughing or sneezing often overcome the supportive strength of these damaged structures, resulting in incontinence. Vaginal delivery, pelvic surgery, hormonal fluctuations, genetic predisposition, and aging are all potential risk factors.

Muscle, fascial, or pudendal nerve injury are potential complications of vaginal delivery.[10] Subsequent atrophy of the rhabdosphincter, levator ani, and fascial support system can occur, resulting in weakening the supportive structures necessary to maintain continence (Figure 2.1).

Although menopause has been recognized by many as a risk factor of SUI, the precise mechanism is unknown. Estrogen receptors are located along the trigone and urethra.[11,12] In these areas estrogen stimulates

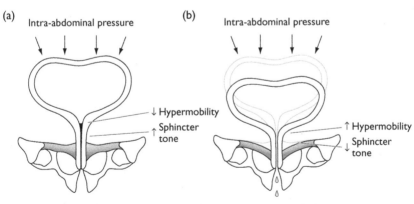

Figure 2.1 Pathophysiology of stress urinary incontinence where (a) continence is maintained and (b) stress urinary incontinence is present.

connective tissue metabolism and collagen production, supporting the theory that estrogen deficiency contributes to atrophy of the supportive tissues of the bladder and urethra, which eventually leads to stress incontinence.[13] A decrease in collagen I, the type of collagen with the greatest tensile strength, has been documented in the arcus tendineus fascia pelvis (ATFP), with menopause.[14] This dense connective tissue represents fascial contributions from the obturator internus and levator ani. The bilateral ATFP bands support the lateral vaginal walls. However, separation of the lateral vaginal walls from the ATFP is the most common site contributing to anterior vaginal prolapse.[15] Chen et al showed that collagen degradation in women with SUI is greater than in continent controls.[16] Addition of in-vitro estrogen produced less response in the incontinent group, suggesting the possibility of genetic differences predisposing patients to SUI.

Thinning of the urethral mucosa can occur due to decreased blood flow associated with a hypoestrogenic state.[17] With ageing, striated muscle atrophy occurs in a predictable pattern at the bladder neck and along the dorsal and ventral walls of the urethra.[18,19] Both age-related processes may explain the associated age-related finding of decreased urethral closure pressures.[20]

The etiology of **urge urinary incontinence** has been theorized as being neurogenic or myogenic. What is not debated is that the intricate mechanisms maintaining continence can be disrupted at many levels, resulting in detrusor overactivity and subsequent urge urinary incontinence. Griffiths proposed that there are potentially many subtypes of detrusor overactivity.[21] As these are better defined, therapy can become more specific and effective.

The *myogenic theory* of urge urinary incontinence argues that intrinsic changes in the smooth muscle cells of the bladder create morphologic changes that result in an overactive bladder. Bladder outlet obstruction from genital prolapse can create detrusor hypertrophy due to increased resistance. Detrusor fibrosis, decreased nerve fiber density, and smooth muscle changes have also been observed.[22] The damaged smooth muscle has diminished coordination of its detrusor contraction due to partial denervation. A urothelial-afferent system has been proposed.[23] With distention of the bladder, the urothelium releases ATP, which then releases a cascade of neurotransmitters, such as acetylcholine. The stimulated muscarinic receptors provide feedback to the brain, interpreted as urinary urgency.

The *neurogenic theory* of urge urinary incontinence proposes that bladder overactivity is caused by damage to the central or peripheral nervous system and results in decreased inhibition of detrusor activity. Regression to primitive bladder reflexes resistant to central inhibition then follows. This may include increased afferent input from the lower urinary tract and enhancement of excitatory transmission of the micturition reflex pathway.[7]

Incontinent older women may have decreased cognitive function and a higher prevalence of hyperreflexia of the lower extremities.[24] A region of the right frontal lobe that is active during voluntary voiding is associated with disorientation and urge incontinence when damaged.[25] Patients with neurologic disorders, such as Parkinson's disease and Alzheimer's disease, often develop incontinence.

Functional incontinence is associated with diseases that impair mobility or cognitive function, creating barriers to continence, despite an intact lower urinary tract. Often, patients with cognitive disorders do not recognize the urge to void and do not void in a socially acceptable manner. Disruption of the central nervous system can result in poor interpretation of the signals of the need to void, resulting in overflow incontinence, or voiding voluntarily in the wrong social situation.

References

1. Sullivan MP, Yalla SV. Physiology of female micturition. Urol Clin North Am 2002;29(3):499–514.
2. Van Arsdalen K, Wein AJ. Physiology of micturition and continence. In: Krane RJ, Siroky MB, eds. Clinical Neuro-Urology, 2nd edn. New York: Little, Brown, 1991:25–82.
3. Wahle GR, Young GPH, Raz S. Anatomy and pathophysiology of pelvic support. In: Raz S, ed. Female Urology, 2nd edn. Philadelphia: WB Saunders, 1996: 57–72.
4. Elbadawi A. Functional anatomy of the organs of micturition. Urol Clin North Am 1996;23:117–210.
5. DeLancey JO. Structural aspects of the extrinsic continence mechanism. Obstet Gynecol 1988;72:296–301.
6. Retzky SS, Rogers RM. Urinary incontinence in women. Clin Symp 1995;47:2–32.
7. de Groat WC. A neurologic basis for the overactive bladder. Urology 1997;50 (Suppl 6A):36–52.
8. Caulfield MP, Birdsall NJM. International Union of Pharmacology. XVII. Classification of muscarinic acetylcholine receptors. Pharmacol Rev 1998;50:279–90.
9. Abrams P, Cardozo L, Fall M, et al. The standardization of terminology of lower urinary tract function: report from the standardization sub-committee of the international continence society. Am J Obstet Gynecol 2002;187(1): 116–26.
10. Persson J, Wolner-Hanssen P, Rydhstroem H. Obstetric risk factors for stress urinary incontinence: a population-based study. Obstet Gynecol 2000;96: 440–5.
11. Griebling TL, Nygaard IE. The role of estrogen replacement therapy in the management of urinary incontinence and urinary tract infection in postmenopausal women. Endocrinol Metab Clin North Am 1997;26:347–60.
12. Zoubina EV, Smith PG. Expression of estrogen receptors alpha and beta by sympathetic ganglion neurons projecting to the proximal urethra of female rats. J Urol 2003;169:382–5.
13. Hendrix SL. Urinary incontinence and menopause: an evidence-based treatment approach. Disease-A-Month 2002;48:622–36.

14. Moalli PA, Talarico LC, Sung VW, et al. Impact of menopause on collagen subtypes in the arcus tendineus fasciae pelvis. Am J Obstet Gynecol 2004; 190(2):620–7.

15. DeLancey JO. Anatomic aspects of vaginal eversion after hysterectomy. Am J Obstet Gynecol 1992;166:1717–28.

16. Chen B, Wen Y, Wang H, et al. Differences in estrogen modulation of tissue inhibitor of matrix metalloproteinase-1 and matrix metalloproteinase-1 expression in cultured fibroblasts from continent and incontinent women. Am J Obstet Gynecol 2003;189(1):59–65.

17. Kevorkian R. Physiology of incontinence. Clin Geriatr Med 2004;20(3): 409–25.

18. Perucchini D, DeLancey JO, Ashton-Miller JA, et al. Age effects on urethral striated muscle II. Anatomic location of muscle loss. Am J Obstet Gynecol 2002;186(3)356–60.

19. Perucchini D, DeLancey JO, Ashton-Miller JA, et al. Age effects on urethral striated muscle I. Changes in number and diameter of striated muscle fibers in the ventral urethra. Am J Obstet Gynecol 2002;186(3):351–5.

20. Rud T, Andersson KE, Asmussen M, et al. Factors maintaining the intraurethral pressure in women. Invest Urol 1980;17:343–7.

21. Griffiths DJ. Discussion: a neurologic basis for the overactive bladder: focus on brain function. Urology 1997;50(Suppl 6A):53.

22. Elbadawi A, Meyer S. Morphometry of the obstructed detrusor. I: review of the issues. Neurourol Urodyn 1989;8:163–72.

23. Anderson KE. Bladder activiation: afferent mechanisms. Urology 2002; 59(Suppl 5A):43–50.

24. Brockelhurst JC, Dillane JB. Studies of the female bladder in old age II. Cystograms in 100 incontinent women. Gerontol Clin 1980;8:306–19.

25. Blok FMB, Willemsen ATM, Holstege G. A PET study on brain control of micturition in humans. Brain 1997;120:111–21.

Chapter 3

Pathophysiology of fecal incontinence

Johann Pfeifer

Introduction

Fecal incontinence is a socially disabling disease. It is associated with reduced personal hygiene and frequently leads to social isolation and loss of self-esteem.[1] Due to personal embarrassment, the true prevalence remains unclear. Symptoms may vary from occasional gas incontinence to minor soiling to gross fecal incontinence of solid stool. The two groups of individuals mostly affected are females and the elderly. It is estimated that 0.5–1.5%[2] of the normal population suffer from fecal incontinence; if soiling is included, the incidence increases to 5%.[3] In geriatric wards, the incidence is as high as 30%; in psychiatric wards, up to 50%.[4] The pathophysiology of this disease is multifactorial and not yet fully understood. While decades ago fecal incontinence was often seen as 'idiopathic', since the advent of physiology testing, major progress has been made in understanding the complexity of this disease. The aim of this chapter is to highlight the various forms of fecal incontinence and to explain possible pathophysiologic mechanisms as a basis for a proper individually tailored treatment.

Definitions

Before discussing anal incontinence it is important to understand the main factors responsible for continence. Stool consistency, capacity and compliance of the rectum, normal reflex patterns like the rectoanal inhibitory reflex, as well as proper sensitivity, and intact pelvic floor and sphincter muscles all help to retain feces in the rectum. Failure of any of these components (Table 3.1) can lead to anal incontinence. For clinical practice, several definitions are used:

Table 3.1 Factors affecting fecal continence

- Stool volume and consistency
- Small bowel transit
- Colon transit
- Distensibility, tone, and capacity of the rectum
- Motility and evacuability of the rectum
- Anorectal angle
- Anorectal sensory and reflex mechanism
- Motility of the anal canal
- Anal canal high-pressure zone

- **Continence:** the ability to defer the urge to defecate until the time and place are convenient.
- **Anal incontinence:** any involuntary leakage of solid or liquid stool or gas.
- **Fecal incontinence:** leakage of liquid or solid stool.
- **Passive incontinence:** if the main problem of incontinence is due to loss of sensation in the anal canal, this is called passive incontinence. Quite often, there is also an internal anal sphincter defect and a low anal resting pressure.
- **Fecal urgency:** the sensation of urgency combined with the inability to defer defecation for more than 5 minutes.
- **Urge fecal incontinence:** withstanding the urge to defecate is impossible, resulting in incontinence episodes. This is usually due to pelvic floor trauma (e.g. obstetric injury) combined with low squeeze pressures.

Physiologic and anatomic basis of continence

Colon

In good health, approximately 1000–1500 ml of fluid enter the colon each day and about 100–150 ml leave as feces. The human continence mechanism is designed to handle delivery of this amount of solid material on a daily basis. Normal humans can also maintain continence for liquid stool, but in some situations, phasic flows of liquid stool can produce urgency and thus overwhelm the continence mechanisms.[5] This means that if a patient suffers from diarrhea of whatever cause, incontinence can occur due to exhaustion of the anal sphincteric mechanism.

Rectum

The rectum is usually empty. When feces enter this organ, the rectum must adjust to the new situation, if rectal emptying should be delayed. This is accomplished by the process of rectal compliance. The rectum has both viscous and elastic properties. The viscous properties of the rectum allow it to accept a distending fecal bolus and at the same time to reduce intraluminal pressure to keep rectal pressures lower than the actual sphincter pressures and therefore avoid incontinence episodes. Elastic properties of the rectum maintain a low pressure while filling. This ability seems to be dependent on an intact intrinsic nervous system and viable muscle cells. For example, rectal compliance is impaired in Hirschsprung's disease, a disease in which the intrinsic nervous system is affected, as well as in chronic rectal ischemia, a disease in which chronic fibrosis leads to a rigid rectal wall.[6]

Pelvic floor

Neuromuscular control has been the subject of considerable investigation and debate in recent decades. Continence may be under voluntary control by the striated muscle of the external anal sphincter, or conversely, by the autonomic nervous system represented by the smooth muscle fibers of the internal anal sphincter. Anatomically, two concentric muscle cylinders comprise the anal sphincter complex. Embryologically, the internal anal sphincter is the continuation of the circular muscle layer of the rectum. That muscle appears later during embryologic development than the striated musculature.[7] Interestingly, most of the time the internal anal sphincter maintains a state of near-maximal contraction.[5] The major reflex response of this muscle due to rectal distention is relaxation.[6] In contrast, the external anal sphincter, a striated muscle outside the internal anal sphincter cylinder, consists of a subcutaneous, a superficial, and a deep portion. This muscle is mainly under voluntary control, and its main reflex response to rectal distention is contraction, to avoid incontinence. The degree of external sphincter contraction varies with alterations in intra-abdominal pressures and posture.[8] Response of the external anal sphincter can be produced by voluntary control, change of posture, rectal distention, increase of intra-abdominal pressure, and anal dilatation. These responses involve several different neural pathways. The practical hint is that failure of response to any of these mentioned stimuli is indicative either of muscle disease or diffuse neurologic disorder.[8]

The innermost portion of the striated levator ani muscle representing the pelvic floor is the puborectalis muscle. This muscle is interesting, as its fibers originate from the backside of the symphysis and then pass posteriorly around the lower portion of the rectum in a U-shape. During contraction of the pelvic floor, this muscle helps to pull the anorectal junction forward and upward, elongating the anal canal and increasing the angulation between the rectum and the anal canal. This tonically contracted sling causes a 90° angulation between the axis of the rectum and the axis of the anal canal. During defecation, the puborectalis muscle relaxes, the angulation straightens, and stool passage is possible.[9]

The neuroanatomy of the sphincters is still not fully understood. Some decades ago, interesting observations were made in patients undergoing sacral resections. Patients with total sacral nerve loss were incontinent. If the sacral nerves S1 and S2 were spared, continence was reduced and there was a loss of ability to discriminate.[10] If all the sacral nerves on one side were amputated, continence was still intact, demonstrating that nerve supply of the sphincter organ is symmetrical. Only the sensitivity in the anal canal on the affected side was reduced.[10]

In-vitro and in-vivo experiments have made a major contribution toward understanding the function and possible types of receptors. It is well known that ganglia cells are sparse in the internal anal sphincter. However, there is an abundance of nerve fibers innervating the smooth muscle cells of the internal anal sphincter and a high concentration of norepinephrine, the sympathetic neurotransmitter. Sympathetic nerve stimulation or application of the neurotransmitter norepinephrine can contract the internal anal sphincter. Thus, 50–85% of the resting tone is produced by this muscle, which is not under voluntary control.[11] Sympathetic blockade by high spinal anaesthesia (Th6–Th12) demonstrated a fall in anal canal tone of 50%.[12] A similar effect was seen when an infusion of phentolamine, an α-adrenoreceptor antagonist, was administered.[13] It was thought that while the sympathetic nerve via the hypogastric nerve is responsible for contraction, the parasympathetic outflow tract is responsible for inhibition of the internal anal sphincter. However, the effect of low spinal anaesthesia (L5–S1) suggests that parasympathetic nerves have little effect on sphincter tone,[12] though muscarinic receptors on or near the smooth internal anal sphincter can cause relaxation.[13]

The somatic pudendal nerve, which arises from the second, third, and fourth sacral nerves, supplies with direct branches the levator ani, the puborectalis muscle, and the external anal sphincter. The latter is mainly supplied by the second sacral nerve root. Receptors for the external sphincter response must lie either near or in the rectal mucosa, because the reflex disappears after application of a topical anaesthetic.[13] Since lesions of the cauda equina abolish the external sphincter reflex, this reflex is mediated through the spinal cord.[8] This is in contrast to the internal anal sphincter, where the reflex can also be seen in patients with lower spinal cord transection.[10]

Physiology of defecation

When stool enters the rectum, the rectal wall will relax, allowing distention and accommodation of the fecal mass. Via a reflex mechanism, contraction of the external anal sphincter followed by brief relaxation of the upper part of the internal anal sphincter prevents fecal leakage. This relaxation is necessary so that stool can come in contact with the sensible epithelium in the transitional zone just above the dentate line to allow discrimination of stool quality (firm, liquid, gas). This sampling reflex can be investigated during anal manometry (rectoanal inhibitory reflex).[14] The short relaxation is followed by a full contraction of the internal anal sphincter. If unwanted, voluntary contraction of the external anal sphincter starts to restore full closure of the sphincter complex by re-catapulting the rectal content into the sigmoid colon. If defecation is convenient, both sphincters relax and contraction in the rectal ampulla evacuates the rectal content.

Etiology of fecal incontinence

Pseudoincontinence

Pseudoincontinence with perineal soiling, frequency, and urgency must be distinguished from true anal incontinence. Soiling can be caused by prolapsing hemorrhoids, condylomata, fistula-in-ano, perianal dermatologic diseases, or poor hygiene. Similarly, rectal frequency and urgency as a result of loss of the rectal reservoir, abnormal rectal compliance, or irritable bowel syndrome can imitate true anal incontinence. Exact history (prior operations), clinical investigation, and proctoscopy will help to exclude pseudoincontinence.

Overflow incontinence

Fecal impaction, a form of severe constipation, is frequently associated with incontinence. Patients with this form of the disease are usually elderly and often suffer from Parkinson's disease or other neurologic or psychiatric diseases.[15] Quite often, anorectal sensation is impaired, compared to age-matched controls.[16] In severe cases, patients lose the ability to contract the external anal sphincter properly, leading to continuous soiling around the anus from the liquid stool which passes around the impacted fecal mass.

Incontinence with a normal pelvic floor

Diarrhea

When the amount of liquid stools and bowel transit time are increased, even in patients with a normally functioning anal sphincter complex, fecal incontinence can occur. Diarrhea may be a consequence of intestinal resection or internal fistula bypassing much of the gastrointestinal tract, inflammatory bowel disease, laxative abuse, autonomic neuropathy, parasitic infections, specific toxins, or other causes.[5]

Cerebral and psychological factors

The function of the voluntary component of anal sphincter activity may be influenced by the central nervous system. It has been demonstrated that during sleep the activity of the whole gut as well as that of the external anal sphincter is reduced.[17] Cann et al reported incontinence episodes during sleep in patients suffering from irritable bowel disease due to overactivity of the intestine during the night.[18] Psychological factors such as depression, lack of motivation, or anxiety may adversely affect the outcome of biofeedback training in patients with fecal incontinence.[19]

Neurotransmission defects

Defecation, as part of normal social behavior, is under conscious control. The upper motor neurons for the voluntary sphincter muscle lie in the parasagittal motor cortex. They communicate with Onuf's nucleus, which is situated in the sacral and gray matter mainly in the S2 and S3 segments of the cord. The frontal cortex is important for the awareness of the need to defecate. Common neurologic diseases affecting the central nervous system such as cerebrovascular accidents, multiple sclerosis, or dementia can all disturb sphincter function. If sphincter function is still intact and anal pressures are normal, reflex defecation will occur but voluntary inhibition is often impaired. Clinically, patients present with urgency and urge incontinence or, due to poor awareness, with incontinence episodes without any prior warning.[1,9,13]

If lower motor neurons are damaged, there will be pelvic floor disturbances (see below). Very often, patients with neurogenic incontinence present with a complex neurologic lesion involving not just the motor but also the sensory pathway. They may present with frequency, urgency, and urge incontinence, indicative of an upper motor neuron lesion. At the same time, sphincter weakness and a sensory deficit may express lower motor neuron damage. Constipation, overflow incontinence, impaired bladder emptying, and impotence may all be symptoms of a complex neurologic disorder.

Incontinence with abnormal pelvic floor

Congenital disorders

Anorectal malformations occur in about 1/5000 births. They may range from imperforate anus to rectal agenesis.[20] We judge imperforate anus as high or low according to the termination of the gut in correlation to the puborectalis sling. Operative procedures may give these patients some kind of motor bowel control but sensory deficits are frequent.

Metabolic disorders

Disorders such as diabetes mellitus may affect continence in various ways. Autonomic neuropathy may lead to diarrhea and incontinence due to increased anorectal motility and transit. Furthermore, peripheral neuropathy with pudendal neuropathy may be a part of or can itself lead to a weak anal sphincter.[1,5,8,13,20]

Neoplastic disorders

Benign tumors such as a large villous adenoma producing copious mucus can lead to soiling. Malignant tumors can also interfere with continence, either by partial obstruction or by direct infiltration into the sphincter muscles.

Degenerative disorders

Incontinence is often seen in the elderly. It can be caused by cerebral degeneration in combination with diminished rectal sensation as well as a weak anal sphincter.

Disorders of the anal sphincter and pelvic floor muscle

Disrupture of the external anal sphincter usually presents as urgency and urge fecal incontinence. A defect in the internal anal sphincter may lead to incontinence independent of additional external sphincter damage.[9] Clinically, soiling and incontinence during sleep can be expected.

OBSTETRIC INJURY

Anal sphincter damage occurring during childbirth is one of the most common causes of incontinence in middle-aged woman[9] (Figure 3.1).

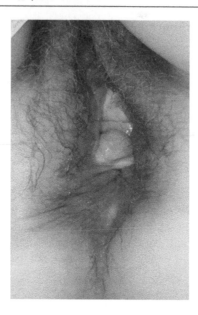

Figure 3.1 Incontinent patient after birth trauma. Note: the perineum is lost. (See also color image on p. xix)

- **External sphincter injury:** occult sphincter defects have been diagnosed in 35% of primiparous women by anal ultrasound.[21] Newer prospective studies confirm the high rate of injuries in vaginal deliveries.[22] Damon et al reported that if there were signs of clinical fecal incontinence and a history of vaginal delivery, endoanal ultrasound would show an anal sphincter defect in 62%.[23] If there have been midline episiotomies and/or operative vaginal delivery, the incidence of sphincter defects increases up to 50%.[24] The gynecologic literature reports the incidence of a third-degree sphincter rupture during vaginal delivery in the normal population as about 2%.[25] The success rate for surgical repair of obstetric sphincter defects is about 75% after 5 years, but it decreases with time, to about 50% after 10 years.[26]
- **Internal sphincter injury:** damage to the internal sphincter may be isolated or in combination with an external sphincter defect. The majority of these defects are anterior.

TRAUMA

Accidental trauma to the sphincter by impalement or gunshot wounds or as a result of a blunt pelvic trauma has been reported.[27] In children, sexual abuse should be excluded; in adults, damage to the sphincter can be the result of retained rectal foreign bodies and anorectal injuries secondary to homosexual activities, sexual assaults, and anal autoeroticism.[28]

SURGERY

Fistula surgery is the most common cause of incontinence due to muscle injuries after operative procedures. Many other operations with more or less extensive grades of anal incontinence have been reported, such as after anal sphincter stretch,[29] hemorrhoidectomy,[10] internal sphincterotomy for chronic anal fissures,[30] and for sphincter-saving operations, for example after coloanal anastomosis for low rectal cancer,[31] or after ilioanal anastomosis with a pouch in patients with ulcerative colitis[32] or familial adenomatous polyposis.[33]

Neurogenic disorders

Neurologic disorders can be classified as cerebral, spinal, and peripheral. The nerves of the pelvic floor can be damaged during childbirth and as a result of excessive straining in constipated patients, leading to stretch injury of the pudendal nerve, which anatomically passes through Alcock's canal to reach the underside of the pelvic floor muscles. Such patients often display physical signs of perineal descent.[34]

PUDENDAL NEUROPATHY

Reduced pudendal nerve conduction velocity frequently induced by deliveries can lead to histologic and physiologic signs of denervation and reinnervation, as proven by pelvic floor electromyography (EMG).[1,5,8,13,20,34] Generally, pudendal nerve function and continence nearly normalize within 6 months after delivery, but neural dysfunction may persist in some patients.[35] Clinically, pudendal neuropathy will lead to low squeeze pressures in the anal canal, an increase in fiber density in the sphincters, and decreased anal canal sensation. However, it must be noted that pudendal neuropathy does not necessarily result in fecal incontinence.[1,5,8,13,20] Prolonged pudendal nerve terminal motor latency measurement may influence the prognosis after surgical corrections of sphincter defects.[36]

AUTONOMIC NEUROPATHY

Reduced sphincter pressures can be a consequence of childbirth. It is hypothesized that autonomic neuropathy may lead to internal sphincter denervation. Although the sphincter looks normal on endoanal ultrasound, low pressures and a poor reflex response are observed.[37] Diabetes, which causes autonomic and somatic neuropathy, may also lead to dysfunction and denervation of both the external and internal anal sphincter.[1,5,8,9,13]

SENSORY IMPAIRMENT AND RECTAL EVACUATION DISORDERS

Disturbed sensation and reduced rectal motility are most often seen in elderly people and there may be clinical signs of overflow incontinence. Another group of patients with sensory difficulties are females with rectoceles.[38,39] Despite intensive efforts to understand the pathophysiology of fecal incontinence, there are still a number of patients whose incontinence remains unexplained, and their disease is still called 'idiopathic fecal incontinence'.

Miscellaneous

AGE

A common form of anal incontinence is that associated with old age. Sphincter pressures as well as cerebral function decrease with age.[14] The precise etiology is often unclear, especially when there is a history of multiparity and concomitant abnormal perineal descent. Furthermore, physical inability to reach the toilet in time can present as fecal incontinence.[40]

RECTAL PROLAPSE

Rectal prolapse is associated with incontinence in about 50% of patients. It is important to differentiate mucus leakage from the prolapse from true incontinence. Factors which are discussed as being responsible for incontinence in these patients are pudendal neuropathy, perineal descent and continuous stretch of the sphincters, and inhibition of the rectoanal inhibitory reflex by the prolapse itself.[41]

RADIATION

Diminished organ nutrition and radiation endarteritis with subsequent atrophy and fibrosis are the result of radiation therapy. Besides sensory deficits, noncompliance of the irradiated rectum is often the biggest problem. When radiation therapy is planned, careful evaluation of the sphincter is recommended and, if function is poor, sphincter-saving procedures should be avoided.[42]

Summary

- Pathophysiologic understanding of the various forms of anal incontinence is a prerequisite for an individual treatment concept.
- The first step is to differentiate between pseudoincontinence, overflow incontinence, and true anal incontinence.

- The next step is to differentiate between incontinence with and without a pelvic floor problem.
- Obstetric sphincter injuries are frequent causes of fecal incontinence.
- Women and elderly patients are most often affected by anal incontinence problems.

References

1. Madoff RD, Parker SC, Varma MG, Lowry AC. Faecal incontinence in adults. Lancet 2004;364:621–32.
2. Mandelstam DA. Faecal incontinence. Social and economic factors. In: Henry MMM, Swash M, eds. Coloproctology and the Pelvic Floor. Pathophysiology and Management. London: Butterworth, 1984:217–22.
3. Drossman DA, Sandler RS, Broom CM, McKee DC. Urgency and fecal soiling in people with bowel dysfunction. Dig Dis Sci 1986;31:1221–5.
4. Thomas TM, Egan M, Walgrove A, Meade TW. The prevalence of fecal and double incontinence. Community Med 1984;6:216–20.
5. Gordon PH. Anal incontinence. In: Gordon PH, Nivatvongs S, eds. Principles and Practice of Surgery for the Colon, Rectum and Anus. St Louis: Quality Medical Publishing, 1992:337–59.
6. Schiller L. Faecal incontinence. Clin Gastroenterol 1986;15:687–701.
7. Levi AC, Borghi F, Garavoglia M. Development of the anal canal muscles. Dis Colon Rectum 1991;34:262–6.
8. Corman ML. Colon and Rectal Surgery, 3rd edn. Philadelphia: JB Lippincott, 1993:188–261.
9. Jorge JM, Wexner SD. Etiology and management of fecal incontinence. Dis Colon Rectum 1993;36:77–97.
10. Stelzner F. Chirurgie an viszeralen Abschlußsystemen. Stuttgart: Georg Thieme Verlag, 1998:121–47.
11. Lestar B, Penninckx F, Kerremans R. The composition of the anal basal pressure. An in vivo and in vitro study in man. Int J Colorectal Dis 1989;4:118–22.
12. Frenckner B, Ihre T. Influence of autonomic nerves on internal anal sphincter in man. Gut 1976;17:306–12.
13. Cook TA, Mortensen N. Colon, rectum, anus, anal sphincters and the pelvic floor. In: Pemberton JH, Swash M, Henry MMM, eds. The Pelvic Floor. Its Function and Disorders. London: WB Saunders, 2002:61–76.
14. Pfeifer J, Oliveira L, Park UC, et al. The relation of normal manometry to age and gender. Techn Coloproctol 1996;4:10–13.
15. Pfeifer J, Agachan F, Wexner SD. Surgery for constipation: a review. Dis Colon Rectum 1996;39:444–60.
16. Read NW, Abouzekry L. Why do patients with faecal impaction have faecal incontinence? Gut 1986;27:283–7.
17. Miller R, Bartolo DCC, Cervero F, Mortensen NJ. Anorectal sampling: a comparison of normal and incontinent patients. Br J Surg 1988;75:44–7.
18. Cann PA, Read NW, Holdsworth CD, Barends D. The role of loperamide and placebo in the management of the irritable bowel syndrome (IBS). Dig Dis Sci 1984;29:239–47.

19. Pager CK, Solomon MJ, Rex J, Roberts RA. Long-term outcomes of pelvic floor exercise and biofeedback treatment for patients with fecal incontinence. Dis Colon Rectum 2002;45:997–1003.
20. Rothenberger DA, Deen KI. Incontinence. In: Nicholls RJ, Dozois RR, eds. Surgery of the Colon and Rectum. New York: Churchill Livingstone, 1997: 739–91.
21. Sultan AH, Kamm MA, Hudson CN, Thomas JM, Bartram CI. Anal-sphincter disruption during vaginal delivery. N Engl J Med 1993;329:1905–11.
22. Zetterstrom J, Mellgren A, Jensen LL, et al. Effect of delivery on anal sphincter morphology and function. Dis Colon Rectum 1999;42:1253–60.
23. Damon H, Henry L, Barth X, Mion F. Fecal incontinence in females with a past history of vaginal delivery: significance of anal sphincter defects detected by ultrasound. Dis Colon Rectum 2002;45:1445–51.
24. Belmonte-Montes C, Hagerman G, Vega-Yepez PA, Hernandez-de-Anda E, Fonseca-Morales V. Anal sphincter injury after vaginal delivery in primiparous females. Dis Colon Rectum 2001;44:1244–8.
25. de Leeuw JW, Struijk PC, Vierhout ME, Wallenburg HC. Risk factors for third degree perineal ruptures during delivery. BJOG 2001;108:383–7.
26. Halverson AL, Hull TL. Long-term outcome of overlapping anal sphincter repair. Dis Colon Rectum 2002;45:345–8.
27. Pfeifer J, Kronberger L, Uranüs S. Injuries to hollow visceral organs. Acta Chir Austrica 1998;6:338–40.
28. Cohen JS, Sackier JM. Management of colorectal foreign bodies. J R Coll Surg Edinb 1996;41:312–15.
29. Goligher JC, Graham NG, Clark CG, De Dombal FT, Giles G. The value of stretching the anal sphincters in the relief of post-haemorrhoidectomy pain. Br J Surg 1969;56:859–61.
30. Mazier P. Keyhole deformity: fact or fiction. Dis Colon Rectum 1985;28:8–10.
31. Williams NS, Price R, Johnson D. The long term effects of sphincter preserving operations for rectal carcinoma on function of the anal sphincter in man. Br J Surg 1980;67:203–8.
32. Rothenberger DA, Vermeulen FD, Christenson CE, et al. Restorative procto-colectomy with ileal reservoir and ileoanal anastomosis. Am J Surg 1983;145:82–8.
33. Ziv Y, Church JM, Oakley JR, et al. Surgery for the teenager with familial adenomatous polyposis: ileo-rectal anastomosis or restorative proctocolectomy? Int J Colorectal Dis 1995;10:6–9.
34. Pfeifer J, Salanga V, Agachan F, Weiss E, Wexner SD. Variation in pudendal nerve terminal motor latency according to disease. Dis Colon Rectum 1997;40:79–83.
35. Ryhammer AM, Laurberg S, Hermann AP. No correlation between perineal position and pudendal nerve terminal motor latency in healthy perimenopausal women. Dis Colon Rectum 1998;41:350–3.
36. Gilliland R, Altomare DF, Moreira H Jr, et al. Pudendal neuropathy is predictive of failure following anterior overlapping sphincteroplasty. Dis Colon Rectum 1998;41:1516–22.
37. Wynne J, Myles J, Jones I, et al. Disturbed anal sphincter function following vaginal delivery. Gut 1996;39:120–4.

38. Heriot AG, Skull A, Kumar D. Functional and physiological outcome following transanal repair of rectocele. Br J Surg 2004;91:1340–4.
39. Sloots CE, Meulen AJ, Felt-Bersma RJ. Rectocele repair improves evacuation and prolapse complaints independent of anorectal function and colonic transit time. Int J Colorectal Dis 2003;18:342–8.
40. Schnelle JF, Leung FW. Urinary and fecal incontinence in nursing homes. Gastroenterology 2004;126(1 Suppl 1):S41–7.
41. Agachan F, Reissman P, Pfeifer J, et al. Comparison of three perineal procedures for the treatment of rectal prolapse. South Med J 1997;90:925–32.
42. Cherry DA, Greenwald ML. Anal incontinence. In: Beck DE, Wexner SD, eds. Fundamentals of Anorectal Surgery. New York: McGraw-Hill, 1992:104–30.

Chapter 4

Pathophysiology of vaginal prolapse

G Willy Davila

Vaginal prolapse, which is the herniation of the bladder, rectum, small intestine, uterus, or other intraperitoneal contents into the vaginal canal, represents a problem of growing public awareness and increasing incidence. Thus, both gynecologists and urologists are caring for an increasing number of patients suffering from symptomatic vaginal prolapse. The recent demographic trend towards the larger number of 'baby-boomers' entering their peri- and postmenopausal years, when incidence of genital prolapse increases, is not an unexpected phenomenon.

It is estimated that approximately 400 000 pelvic reconstructive and anti-incontinence surgeries are performed in the United States on a yearly basis. This number will probably continue to increase, as it is estimated that 11% of women will need an operation for prolapse or incontinence with a 30% reoperation rate.[1] For a reconstructive surgeon, a clear understanding of anatomic alterations leading to the development of genital prolapse is of crucial importance. Surgical therapy directed at correction of specific anatomic defects will only be effective if the surgeon is keenly aware of the underlying anatomic alterations and performs the right procedure for each segmental prolapse. This is of special importance in the treatment of vaginal vault prolapse, which in a post-hysterectomy patient can present with rather subtle findings.

Pathophysiology

Underlying most forms of pelvic floor dysfunction is direct tissue damage resultant from passage of a relatively large fetus through a relatively small vaginal hiatus during the vaginal birth process. Weakening muscular support of the pelvic floor due to neuromuscular injury from a vaginal delivery will lead to perineal and pelvic floor descent and marked strain on supporting ligaments and connective tissue. Specific tears and the supporting infrastructure of the pelvic structures also occur during the vaginal delivery process. These include separation of lateral vaginal support from the pelvic sidewall as well as tearing of superior uterine support along the uterosacral ligament/cardinal ligament complex. Complete avoidance of the vaginal delivery process may not be completely protective, as pregnancy itself has been noted to result in significant strain on the pelvic floor supporting structure. Although a primary cesarean section may protect from most forms of pelvic floor dysfunction, it has been estimated that three unlabored cesarean sections may result in a similar impact as one vaginal delivery. In addition, chronic increases in intra-abdominal pressure – such as chronic coughing, chronic constipation, and other physical activities associated with increased Valsalva efforts – may lead to weakening of pelvic support structures. Genetic connective tissue weakness and postmenopausal estrogen-deficiency-related urogenital atrophy can also promote development of genital prolapse.

Normal anatomic support

In order for pelvic anatomy to be maintained, appropriate support must be present along the vaginal apex, perineal body, and the intervening anterior and posterior vaginal walls. The different areas of support are illustrated in Figure 4.1.

Apical support

The uterine cervix provides a focal point for attachment of the uterosacral and cardinal ligaments. These are primarily responsible for apical support by attachment vertically towards the sacrum (uterosacral ligaments) and laterally (cardinal ligaments) towards the ischial spines.[2] In cervical/uterine prolapse, the cervix either becomes detached from the ligament complex or there is significant hypertrophy of the cervix with maintenance of good vault support (Figure 4.2). This is an important differentiation when evaluating a patient with uterine prolapse. If the patient has isolated cervical hypertrophy (which can lead to a cervix of 8–10 cm in length) without apical prolapse, surgery will entail a simple hysterectomy or Manchester procedure associated with cervical amputation. However, if uterine prolapse without cervical hypertrophy is found, it will probably be associated with posterior weakness of apical support and require performance of a McCall's or Mayo culdoplasty to restore vaginal support to the proximal uterosacral ligaments (Figure 4.3). Preoperative examination is therefore crucial in assessing the anatomy associated with cervical prolapse.

In a post-hysterectomy patient, either cardinal or uterosacral ligaments can become detached from the vaginal apex, resulting in apical prolapse (Figure 4.4). This emphasizes the importance of reattachment of the ligaments to the cuff at the time of hysterectomy. Various techniques are clinically used to reattach the ligaments to the apex at the time of hysterectomy but are not universally utilized by gynecologic surgeons. Besides removal of

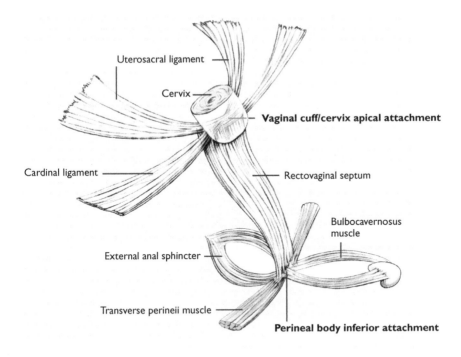

Uterosacral ligament

Cervix

Vaginal cuff/cervix apical attachment

Cardinal ligament

Rectovaginal septum

Bulbocavernosus muscle

External anal sphincter

Transverse perineii muscle

Perineal body inferior attachment

Figure 4.1 Normal vaginal support anatomy with interconnected apical support (cardinal and uterosacral ligaments), posterior wall fibromuscular endopelvic fascia, and the perineal body musculature.

the uterus, the principal focus at the time of a hysterectomy (especially for prolapse) should be in restoration of vault support with a McCall or Mayo culdoplasty designed to reattach the uterosacral and cardinal ligaments to the vaginal cuff. Post-hysterectomy vault prolapse can be effectively prevented with these techniques (see Ch. 13).

When post-hysterectomy vaginal vault prolapse occurs, it is of crucial importance for the reconstructive surgeon to recognize this anatomic alteration during the preoperative evaluation. During physical examination, there will typically be a transverse band of scar tissue visible at the apex with a 'dimple' at either end of the scar band. These dimples represent previous attachment sites of the uterosacral and cardinal ligaments and are a very useful landmark for identification of vault prolapse.[3] In a traditional culdoplasty, surgical therapy is directed at restoring connection of the vaginal apex to the uterosacral ligaments intraoperatively. Recent trends have been directed at recreating ligamentous support utilizing synthetic tapes or performing the suspension to clearly identifiable uterosacral ligaments

(a)

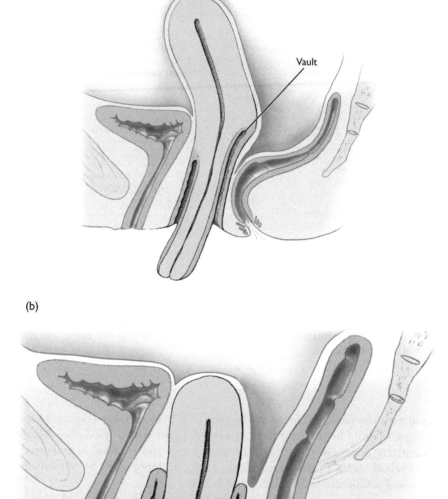

Vault

(b)

Figure 4.2 Uterine/cervical prolapse can be present as isolated cervical hypertrophy without apical prolapse (a), apical prolapse without cervical hypertrophy (b), or a combination of both.

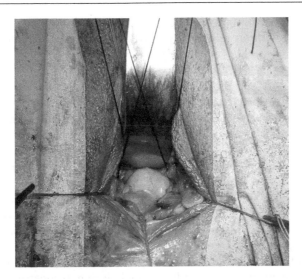

Figure 4.3 A McCall culdoplasty incorporates both uterosacral ligaments, intervening posterior cul-de-sac peritoneum, and full thickness of the apical vaginal wall. (See also color image on p. xix)

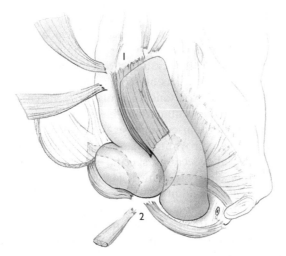

Figure 4.4 Prolapse can develop as a consequence of separation of the uterosacral or cardinal ligaments apically, fibromuscular layer anteriorly or posteriorly, or the perineal body musculature. 1. Vaginal apex with separated attachments of uterosacral and cardinal ligaments. 2. Perineal body with separated attachments of bulbocavernosus, transverse perineii, and external anal sphincter muscles.

laparoscopically. Alternatively, other forms of vault suspension techniques are performed without utilizing the endogenous support ligaments.

Perineal anatomy

The inferior-most pelvic support is localized at the perineal body, between the anus and the vagina. This structure represents a condensation of connective and muscular tissue, including the anterior attachment of the external anal sphincter, medial attachment of the transverse perineii muscles, and posterior attachment of the bulbocavernosus muscles (Figure 4.1). This condensation forms a fulcrum of attachment of these muscles as well as of the fibromuscular tissue entailing the rectovaginal septum fascia. The perineal body begins at the level of the levator musculature and extends down to the perineal skin. Muscular weakness and development of tears along the perineal body will lead to perineal descent, placing further strain on apical supports and thus further anatomic support weakness. Restoration of perineal body integrity is frequently ignored during reconstructive surgery, resulting in incomplete restoration of anatomy and jeopardizing a surgical repair. The muscles that form the perineal body are not easily identified during surgical dissection. They typically represent a condensation of connective tissue that is deficient in most women with advanced prolapse.

Fibromuscular (fascial) support structures

A layer of fibromuscular tissue, more commonly known as 'fascia', surrounds the entire vaginal canal. This endopelvic fascia has traditionally been dissected free from the overlying vaginal epithelium and then plicated in the midline in order to correct a cystocele or rectocele. Further understanding of the role of this fascia has allowed us to improve our surgical techniques as well as clarify the reasons for prolapse recurrence and surgical failures. Recent histologic examinations have determined that endopelvic fascia is truly a fibromuscular layer.[4] As such, its strength is debatable, and thus its role in providing anatomic support is controversial. Nevertheless, during surgical dissections, specific detachments or tears in the fibromuscular layer can be clearly identified. These defects have been popularized as 'site-specific tears'. In addition, correction of site-specific tears or separations from normal support structures has satisfactorily restored anatomic support in many patients. Thus, although controversy persists, there is certainly an important role for the vaginal wall fibromuscular layer in providing normal anatomic support.

The fibromuscular layer along the anterior vaginal wall is known as the pubocervical fascia. Posteriorly, it is known as the rectovaginal septum, or Denonvilliers' fascia. This posterior fascia has primarily been described in males, but is also present in females as a layer of fibromuscular tissue from the perineal body to the vaginal apex or cervix. It is thus important to recognize that the entire vaginal canal is enveloped by intact fascia with attachments apically, inferiorly, and laterally. Tears in the fibromuscular layer can develop at either of the attachment sites or within the layer itself. Separations of endopelvic fascia from its lateral attachments are known as *paravaginal defects* and typically lead to cystocele development. Paravaginal detachments are most commonly found on the right side. Work by anatomists on fresh cadavers demonstrated the high incidence of paravaginal defects in women, and led to the popularity of paravaginal defect repairs. However, this popularity for correction of cystoceles has declined, as surgeons have begun to realize that paravaginal defects do not always need to be repaired. In addition, correction of a paravaginal defect may require an abdominal procedure or a tedious vaginal repair.

Recently, our understanding of the frequency of fascial tears has improved with intraoperative dissection. Careful examination of prolapse segments as well as careful dissection of the fibromuscular layer from the overlying vaginal epithelium frequently identifies specific tears in this fibromuscular layer. It has become clear that fascial tears tend to begin as apical transverse defects, or separation of the fibromuscular layer from the vaginal apex or cervix, with the highest degree of frequency. Recent studies from our center reveal that the highest incidence of fascial separation occurs as superior transverse fascial defects posteriorly.[5] This will typically lead to the formation of what is commonly thought of as an enterocele. Restoration of attachment of this layer to the vaginal apex will most often also reduce an obvious rectocele. Thus, restoration of intact attachment of the fibromuscular layer to the vaginal cuff can be an important part of the correction of any posterior vaginal prolapse. Along the anterior vaginal wall, superior transverse fibromuscular layer separation is also very common in the development of a cystocele, and may be more clinically significant than paravaginal separation.[4]

Inferior perineal defects were thought to be quite common, especially in posterior wall prolapse. Our experience has shown that although they do exist, their frequency is not as high as that of superior transverse defects.

The frequent difficulty in identifying specific fascial defects has led to the increasing popularity of biologic and synthetic grafts in reconstructive surgery. Under currently utilized techniques, a graft is utilized to reinforce and/or replace endogenous endopelvic fibromuscular tissue. If attached from sidewall to sidewall and from apex to perineum, the usage of a graft would in fact obviate the need for correction of specific defects or tears.

Neuromuscular function

It is well understood that appropriate function of the levator musculature is required for appropriate pelvic support as well as pelvic visceral function.

Injury to the pudendal nerves and/or direct injury to the levator muscles will lead to weakness and descent of the levator plate, resulting in enlargement of the levator hiatus and increasing propensity to prolapse of the pelvic organs. In women with significant pelvic neuropathy, the levator muscles assume a more vertical configuration as compared to a conical figuration, thus resulting in worsening support of pelvic structures. During reconstructive surgery, restoration of muscular support is very important. Although levator plication is controversial due to the increased risk of dyspareunia, this procedure in fact may help normalize muscular support to the pelvis.

Conclusions

Genital prolapse develops as a consequence of multiple factors, including weakness in the endopelvic fibromuscular layer, neuromuscular dysfunction of the pelvic floor, and tears along ligament support structures. Surgical treatment of genital prolapse is based on accurate identification of the prolapsed segment as well as the anatomic defect responsible for that prolapse. Current trends in surgical practice are focused on correcting specific support defects. Future trends in surgical reconstruction are directed towards comprehensive pelvic floor reconstruction with grafts to correct multiple defects simultaneously.

References

1.   Olsen AL, Smith VJ, Bergstrom JO, Colling JC, Clark AL. Epidemiology of surgically managed pelvic organ prolapse and urinary incontinence. Obstet Gynecol 1997;89(4):501–6.
2.   Davila GW. Vaginal vault surgery. In: Pelvic Floor Dysfunction: A Multidisciplinary Approach. Davila GW, Wexner SD and Ghoniem GM, eds. Springer-Verlag, London, 2005.
3.   Biller D, Davila GW. Choosing the best technique for vaginal vault prolapse. OBG Management 2004;16(12):21–34.
4.   Weber AM, Walters MD. Anterior vaginal prolapse: review of anatomy and techniques of surgical repair. Obstet Gynecol 1997; 89:331–8.
5.   Guerette N, Davila GW. Can discrete vaginal fascial defects be accurately identified preoperatively? Neurourol Urodyn 2004;23(5/6):436–437.

Chapter 5

Estrogens and the urogenital tract

Dudley Robinson and Linda Cardozo

Introduction

The female genital and lower urinary tract share a common embryologic origin from the urogenital sinus (Figure 5.1) and both are sensitive to the effects of female sex steroid hormones.

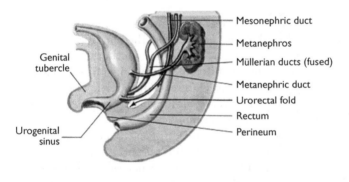

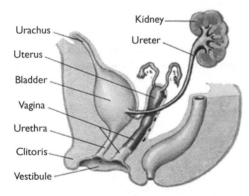

Figure 5.1 Embryologic origin of the female genital and lower urinary tract. (See also color image on p. xx)

Estrogen is known to have an important role in the function of the lower urinary tract throughout adult life, and estrogen and progesterone receptors have been demonstrated in the vagina, urethra, bladder, and pelvic floor musculature.[1-4] Estrogen deficiency that occurs following menopause is known to cause atrophic changes within the urogenital tract[5] and is associated with urinary symptoms such as frequency, urgency, nocturia, incontinence, and recurrent infection. These may coexist with symptoms of vaginal atrophy such as dyspareunia, itching, burning, and dryness.

Estrogen receptors

The effects of the steroid hormone 17β-estradiol (Figure 5.2) are mediated by ligand-activated transcription factors known as estrogen receptors, which are glycoproteins sharing common features with androgen and progesterone receptors.

The classic estrogen receptor (ERα) was first discovered by Elwood Jensen in 1958 and cloned from uterine tissue in 1986,[6] although it was not until 1996 that the second estrogen receptor (ERβ) was identified[7] (Figure 5.3).

Estrogen receptors have been demonstrated throughout the lower urinary tract and are expressed in the squamous epithelium of the proximal and distal urethra, vagina, and trigone of the bladder,[8] although not in the dome of the bladder, reflecting its different embryologic origin (Figure 5.4). The pubococcygeous and the musculature of the pelvic floor have also been shown to be estrogen-sensitive,[9,10] although estrogen receptors have not yet been identified in the levator ani muscles.[11]

More recently, the distribution of estrogen receptors throughout the urogenital tract has been studied, with both α and β receptors being found in the vaginal walls and uterosacral ligaments of premenopausal women, although the latter was absent in the vaginal walls of postmenopausal women.[12] In addition, α receptors are localized in the urethral sphincter, and when sensitized by estrogens, are thought to help maintain muscular tone.[13] Interestingly, estrogen receptors have also been identified in mast cells in women with interstitial cystitis[14] and in the male lower urinary tract.

Figure 5.2 Estrogen molecule.

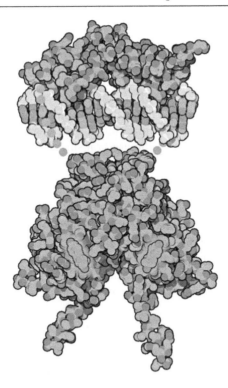

Figure 5.3 Estrogen receptor from the Molecule of the Month series by David S. Goodsell of The Scripps Research Institute http://www.rcsb.org/pdb/molecules/pdb45_1.html. (See also color image on p. xxi)

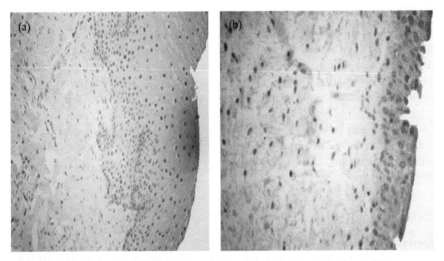

Figure 5.4 Estrogen receptors (stained dark blue) are present in the subepithelium of the vagina (a), although they have much lower expression in the bladder (b). (See also color image on p. xxi)

Lower urinary tract function

Estrogens play an important role in the continence mechanism, with bladder and urethral function becoming less efficient with age.[15] Elderly women have been found to have a reduced flow rate, increased urinary residuals, higher filling pressures, reduced bladder capacity, and lower maximum voiding pressures.[16] Estrogens may affect continence by increasing urethral resistance, raising the sensory threshold of the bladder, or by increasing α-adrenoreceptor sensitivity in the urethral smooth muscle.[17,18]

Bladder function

Estrogen is known to have a direct effect on detrusor function through modifications in muscarinic receptors[19,20] and by inhibition of movement of extracellular calcium ions into muscle cells.[21] Consequently, estradiol has been shown to reduce the amplitude and frequency of spontaneous rhythmic detrusor contractions;[22] there is also evidence that it may increase the sensory threshold of the bladder in some women.[23]

Neurologic control

Sex hormones are known to influence the central neurologic control of micturition, although their exact role in the micturition pathway has yet to be elucidated. Estrogen receptors have been demonstrated in the cerebral cortex, limbic system, hippocampus, and cerebellum.[24,25]

Urethra

Estrogen receptors have been demonstrated in the squamous epithelium of both the proximal and distal urethra,[24] and estrogen has been shown to improve the maturation index of urethral squamous epithelium.[26] It has been suggested that estrogen increases urethral closure pressure and improves pressure transmission to the proximal urethra, both promoting continence.[27–30] The vascular pulsations seen on urethral pressure profilometry secondary to blood flow in the urethral submucosa and urethral sphincter have been shown to increase in size following estrogen administration,[31] whereas the effect is lost following estrogen withdrawal at menopause.

Collagen

Estrogens are known to have an effect on collagen synthesis (Figure 5.5) and they have been shown to have a direct effect on collagen metabolism in the lower genital tract.[32] Changes found in women with urogenital atrophy

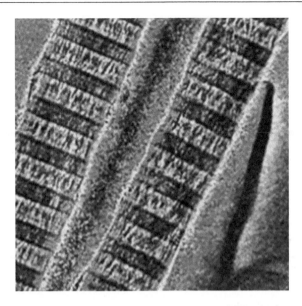

Figure 5.5 Scanning electron micrograph of collagen fibers. Each is composed of three chains wound together in a triple helix.

may represent an alteration in systemic collagenase activity,[33] and urodynamic stress incontinence and urogenital prolapse have been associated with a reduction in both vaginal and periurethral collagen.[34-36]

Urogenital atrophy

Withdrawal of endogenous estrogen at menopause results in climacteric symptoms such as hot flushes and night sweats in addition to the less commonly reported symptoms of urogenital atrophy. Symptoms do not usually develop until several years following the menopause when levels of endogenous estrogens fall below the level required to promote endometrial growth.[37] This temporal relationship would suggest estrogen withdrawal as the cause.

Vaginal dryness is commonly the first reported symptom and is caused by a reduction in mucus production within the vaginal glands (Table 5.1). The signs associated with urogenital atrophy are listed in Table 5.2.

Atrophy within the vaginal epithelium leads to thinning and an increased susceptibility to infection and mechanical trauma (Figure 5.6). Glycogen depletion within the vaginal mucosa following menopause leads to a decrease in lactic acid formation by Döderlein's lactobacillus and a consequent rise in vaginal pH from around 4 to between 6 and 7. This allows

Table 5.1 Symptoms of urogenital atrophy

Vaginal dryness

Dyspareunia

Vaginal burning

Pruritis

Urinary symptoms: urgency, frequency, nocturia, dysuria, recurrent infection

Prolapse

Table 5.2 Signs of urogenital atrophy

Pallor/inflammation

Petechiae

Epithelial or mucosal thinning

Decreased elasticity

Urogenital prolapse

bacterial overgrowth and colonization with Gram-negative bacilli, compounding the effects of vaginal atrophy and leading to symptoms of vaginitis such as pruritus, dyspareunia, and discharge (Figure 5.7). In order to clinically grade and quantify the changes associated with urogenital atrophy, a scoring system has been developed based on a five-point scale[38] (Table 5.3).

Lower urinary tract symptoms

Epidemiologic studies have implicated estrogen deficiency in the etiology of lower urinary tract symptoms, with 70% of women relating the onset of urinary incontinence to their final menstrual period.[5] Urge incontinence, in particular, is more prevalent following menopause, and the prevalence would appear to rise with increasing years of estrogen deficiency.[39] There is, however, conflicting evidence regarding the role of estrogen withdrawal at the time of the menopause. Some studies have shown a peak incidence in perimenopausal women,[40,41] whereas other evidence suggests that many women develop incontinence at least 10 years prior to the cessation of

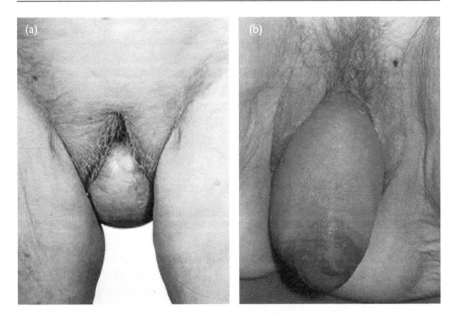

Figure 5.6 Vaginal vault prolapse (a) and third-degree uterine prolapse (b) in postmenopausal women complaining of urogenital atrophy. (See also color image on p. xxii)

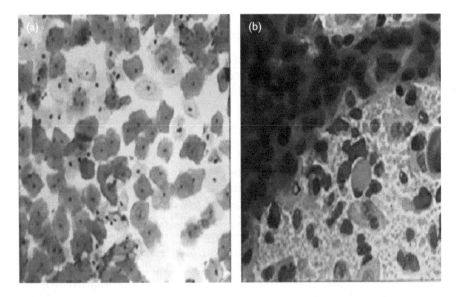

Figure 5.7 Vaginal cytology in a healthy premenopausal woman (a) and following the menopause in a woman with symptomatic vaginal atrophy (b). (See also color image on p. xxii)

Table 5.3 The vaginal health index

Overall elasticity

Fluid secretion (type and consistency)

pH

Epithelial integrity

Moisture

---

menstruation, with significantly more premenopausal women than post-menopausal women affected.[42]

Urinary tract infection is also a common cause of urinary symptoms in women of all ages. This is a particular problem in the elderly, with a reported incidence of 20% in the community and over 50% in institutionalized patients.[43,44] Pathophysiologic changes, such as impairment of bladder emptying, poor perineal hygiene and both fecal and urinary incontinence, may partly account for the high prevalence observed. In addition, changes in the vaginal flora due to estrogen depletion lead to colonization with Gram-negative bacilli, which in addition to causing local irritative symptoms, also act as uropathogens.

Estrogens in the management of incontinence

Estrogen preparations have been used for many years in the treatment of urinary incontinence,[45,46] although their precise role remains controversial. Many of the studies performed have been uncontrolled observational series that have examined the use of a wide range of different preparations, doses, and routes of administration. The inconsistent use of progestogens to provide endometrial protection is a further confounding factor that makes interpretation of the results difficult.

In order to clarify the situation, a meta-analysis from the HUT Committee was reported.[47] Of 166 articles identified, which were published in English between 1969 and 1992, only 6 were controlled trials and 17 were uncontrolled series. Meta-analysis found an overall significant effect of estrogen therapy on subjective improvement in all subjects and for subjects with urodynamic stress incontinence alone. Subjective improvement rates with estrogen therapy in randomized controlled trials ranged from 64% to 75%, although placebo groups also reported an improvement of 10–56%. In uncontrolled series, subjective improvement rates were 8–89%, whereas subjects with urodynamic stress incontinence showed improvement of 34–73%. However, when assessing objective fluid loss, there was no significant effect. Maximum urethral closure pressure was found to increase significantly with estrogen therapy, although this outcome was influenced by a single study showing a large effect.[48]

A further meta-analysis performed in Italy has analyzed the results of randomized controlled clinical trials on the efficacy of estrogen treatment in postmenopausal women with urinary incontinence.[49] A search of the literature (1965–1996) revealed 72 articles, of which only four met the meta-analysis criteria. There was a statistically significant difference in subjective outcome between estrogen and placebo, although there was no such difference in objective or urodynamic outcome. The authors conclude that this difference could be relevant, although the studies may have lacked objective sensitivity to detect this.

The role of estrogen replacement therapy in the prevention of ischemic heart disease has recently been assessed in a 4-year randomized trial, the Heart and Estrogen/progestin Replacement Study (HERS)[50] involving 2763 postmenopausal women younger than 80 years old with intact uteri and ischemic heart disease. In the study, 55% of women reported at least one episode of urinary incontinence each week and were randomly assigned to oral conjugated estrogen plus medroxyprogesterone acetate or placebo daily. Incontinence improved in 26% of women assigned to placebo as compared to 21% receiving hormone replacement therapy (HRT), whereas 27% of the placebo group complained of worsening symptoms compared with 39% in the HRT group ($p = 0.001$). The incidence of incontinent episodes per week increased an average of 0.7 in the HRT group and decreased by 0.1 in the placebo group ($p < 0.001$). Overall, combined hormone replacement therapy was associated with worsening stress and urge urinary incontinence, although there was no significant difference in daytime frequency, nocturia, or number of urinary tract infections.

These findings have also been confirmed in the Nurse's Health Study which followed 39 436 postmenopausal women aged 50–75 years old over a 4-year period. The risk of incontinence was found to be elevated in those women taking HRT when compared to those who had never taken HRT. There was an increase in risk in women taking oral estrogen (RR = 1.54; 95% CI 1.44–1.65), transdermal estrogen (RR = 1.68; 95% CI 1.41–2.00), oral estrogen and progesterone (RR = 1.34; 95% CI 1.24–1.34), and transdermal estrogen and progesterone (RR = 1.46; CI 1.16–1.84). In addition, while there remained a small risk after the cessation of HRT (RR = 1.14; 95% CI 1.06–1.23), by 10 years the risk was identical (RR = 1.02; 95% CI 0.91–1.41) and was identical to those women who had never taken HRT.[51]

More recently, the effects of oral estrogens and progestogens on the lower urinary tract have been assessed in 32 female nursing home residents,[52] with an average age of 88 years. Subjects were randomized to oral estrogen and progesterone or placebo for 6 months. At follow-up, there was no difference between severity of incontinence, prevalence of bacteriuria, or the results of vaginal cultures, although there was an improvement in atrophic vaginitis in the placebo group.

The most recent meta-analysis of the effect of estrogen therapy on the lower urinary tract has been performed by the Cochrane group.[53] Overall, 28 trials were identified, including 2926 women. In the 15 trials comparing estrogen to placebo, there was a higher subjective impression of improvement rate in those women taking estrogen, and this was the case for all types of incontinence (RR for cure = 1.61; 95% CI 1.04–2.49). Equally, when subjective cure and improvement were taken together, there was a statistically higher cure and improvement rate for both urge (57% vs 28%) and stress (43% vs 27%) incontinence. In those women with urge incontinence, the chance of improvement was 25% higher than in women with stress incontinence and, overall, about 50% of women treated with estrogen were cured or improved compared with 25% on placebo. The authors concluded that estrogens can improve or cure incontinence and that the effect may be most useful in women complaining of urge incontinence.

Estrogens in the management of stress incontinence

In addition to the studies included in the HUT meta-analysis, several authors have also investigated the role of estrogen therapy in the management of urodynamic stress incontinence only. Oral estrogens have been reported to increase the maximum urethral pressures and lead to symptomatic improvement in 65–70% of women,[54,55] although other work has not confirmed this.[56,57] More recently, two placebo-controlled studies have been performed examining the use of oral estrogens in the treatment of urodynamic stress incontinence in postmenopausal women. Neither conjugated equine estrogens and medroxyprogesterone,[58] or unopposed estradiol valerate[59] showed a significant difference in either subjective or objective outcomes. Furthermore, a review of 8 controlled and 14 uncontrolled prospective trials concluded that estrogen therapy was not an efficacious treatment for stress incontinence but may be useful for symptoms of urgency and frequency.[60]

A recently reported meta-analysis has helped determine the role of estrogen replacement in women with stress incontinence.[61] Of the papers reviewed, 14 were non-randomized studies, six randomized trials (of which four were placebo controlled), and two meta-analyses. Interestingly, there was only a symptomatic or clinical improvement noted in the nonrandomized studies, whereas no such effect was noted in the randomized trials. The authors conclude that, currently, the evidence would not support the use of estrogen replacement alone in the management of stress incontinence.

Estrogens in the management of urge incontinence

Estrogens have been used in the treatment of urinary urgency and urge incontinence for many years, although there have been few controlled trials to confirm their efficacy. A double-blind placebo-controlled crossover study using oral estriol in 34 postmenopausal women produced subjective improvement in 8 women with mixed incontinence and 12 with urge incontinence.[62] However, a double-blinded multicenter study of the use of estriol (3 mg/day) in postmenopausal women complaining of urgency has failed to confirm these findings,[63] showing both subjective and objective improvement, but with no significant improvement over placebo. Estriol is a naturally occurring weak estrogen, which has little effect on the endometrium and does not prevent osteoporosis, although it has been used in the treatment of urogenital atrophy. Consequently, it is possible that the dosage or route of administration in this study was not appropriate in the treatment of urinary symptoms, and higher systemic levels may be required.

The use of sustained-release 17β-estradiol vaginal tablets (Vagifem, Novo Nordisk) (Figure 5.8) has also been examined in postmenopausal women with urgency and urge incontinence or urodynamic diagnosis of sensory urgency or detrusor overactivity. Following a 6-month course of treatment, the only significant difference between the active and placebo groups was an improvement in the symptom of urgency in those women with a urodynamic diagnosis of sensory urgency.[64] A further double-blinded, randomized, placebo-controlled trial of vaginal 17β-estradiol vaginal tablets has shown lower urinary tract symptoms of frequency, urgency, and urge and stress incontinence to be significantly improved, although there was no objective urodynamic assessment performed.[65] In both of these studies, the subjective improvement in symptoms may simply represent local estrogenic effects reversing urogenital atrophy rather than a direct effect on bladder function.

To try and clarify the role of estrogen therapy in the management of women with urge incontinence, a meta-analysis of the use of estrogen in women with symptoms of overactive bladder has been reported by the HUT Committee (unpublished work). In a review of 10 randomized placebo-controlled trials, estrogen was found to be superior to placebo when considering symptoms of urge incontinence, frequency, and nocturia, although vaginal estrogen administration was found to be superior for symptoms of urgency. In those patients taking estrogens, there was also a significant increase in first sensation and bladder capacity compared with those taking placebo.

In one study, the researchers recruited more than 27 347 postmenopausal women, aged 50–79 years old, who were enrolled in the National Institutes of Health-sponsored Women's Health Initiative between 1993 and 1998.[66]

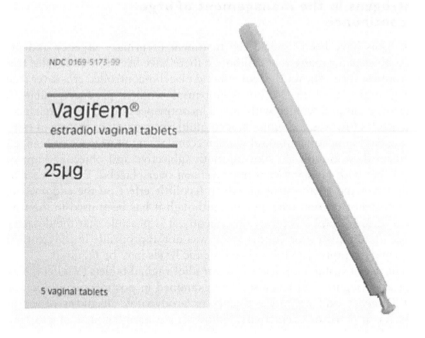

Figure 5.8 Vagifem tablets, pack and applicator.

The subjects were randomized based on hysterectomy status to receive (following a 3-month 'washout' period) either (1) estrogen alone (5310 women); (2) estrogen plus progestin (8506 women), or (3) placebo (5429 women).

Among the researchers' findings at 1 year:

- HRT in general increased the incidence of all types of urinary incontinence (UI);
- the risk was highest for stress UI;
- combination estrogen and progestin therapy had no effect on developing urge UI;
- among women experiencing UI at baseline, frequency worsened for subjects receiving estrogen alone as well as those receiving estrogen plus progestin.

Based on their analysis, the researchers concluded that, at 1 year, HRT with either estrogen alone or estrogen plus progestin increased the risk of UI among continent women and worsened the symptoms of those with the condition at baseline. Based on these findings, the authors recommend that clinicians should no longer prescribe long-term oral conjugated equine estrogens for treatment of urge, stress, or mixed UI in postmenopausal women aged 50 years old or older. However, whether topical estrogens might prove beneficial remains unknown, especially on a short-term basis and/or in combination with other therapies.

Estrogens in the management of recurrent urinary tract infection

Estrogen therapy has been shown to increase vaginal pH and reverse the microbiologic changes that occur in the vagina following the menopause.[67] Initial small, uncontrolled studies using oral or vaginal estrogens in the treatment of recurrent urinary tract infection appeared to give promising results[68,69] although unfortunately this has not been supported by larger randomized trials.

Kjaergaard and colleagues[70] compared vaginal estriol tablets with placebo in 21 postmenopausal women over a 5-month period and found no significant difference between the two groups. However, a subsequent randomized, double-blind placebo-controlled study assessing the use of estriol vaginal cream in 93 postmenopausal women during an 8-month period did reveal a significant effect.[71]

Kirkengen et al randomized 40 postmenopausal women to receive either placebo or oral estriol and found that although initially both groups had a significantly decreased incidence of recurrent infections, after 12 weeks estriol was shown to be significantly more effective.[72] However, these findings were not confirmed in a subsequent trial of 72 postmenopausal women with recurrent urinary tract infections randomized to oral estriol or placebo. Following a six-month treatment period and a further 6-month follow-up, estriol was found to be no more effective than placebo.[73]

More recently, a randomized, open, parallel-group study assessing the use of an estradiol-releasing silicone vaginal ring (Estring; Pharmacia and Upjohn, Sweden) (Figure 5.9) in postmenopausal women with recurrent infections has been performed, which showed the cumulative likelihood of remaining infection free was 45% in the active group and 20% in the placebo group.[74] Estring was also shown to decrease the number of recurrences per year and to prolong the interval between infection episodes.

Estrogens in the management of urogenital atrophy

Symptoms of urogenital atrophy do not occur until the level of endogenous estrogen is lower than that required to promote endometrial proliferation. Consequently, it is possible to use a low dose of estrogen replacement therapy in order to alleviate urogenital symptoms while avoiding the risk of

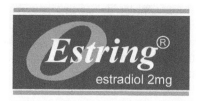

2 mg
estradiol
afgifte: ca 7.5ug /24 uur

1 vaginale ring

Figure 5.9 Estring estradiol ring.

endometrial proliferation and removing the necessity of providing endo-metrial protection with progestogens.[75] The dose of estradiol commonly used in systemic estrogen replacement is usually 25–100 µg, although studies investigating the use of estrogens in the management of urogenital symp-toms have shown that 8–10 µg of vaginal estradiol is effective.[76] Thus, only 10–30% of the dose used to treat vasomotor symptoms may be effective in the management of urogenital symptoms. Since 10–25% of women receiving systemic HRT still experience the symptoms of urogenital atrophy,[77] low-dose local preparations may have an additional beneficial effect (Table 5.4).

A recent review of estrogen therapy in the management of urogenital atrophy has been performed by the HUT Committee.[78] Ten randomized tri-als and 54 uncontrolled series were examined from 1969 to 1995, assessing 24 different treatment regimens. Meta-analysis of 10 placebo-controlled trials confirmed the significant effect of estrogens in the management of urogenital atrophy.

Table 5.4 Vaginal estrogen preparations

Type of estrogen	Mode of administration	
Estriol	Cream:	**Ovestin**
	Pessary:	**Orthogynest**
Estradiol	Tablets:	**Vagifem**
	Ring:	**Estring**
Conjugated	Cream:	**Premarin**

The route of administration was assessed, and oral, vaginal, and parenteral (transcutaneous patches and subcutaneous implants) routes were compared. Overall, the vaginal route of administration was found to correlate with better symptom relief, greater improvement in cytologic findings, and higher serum estradiol levels.

With regard to the type of estrogen preparation, estradiol was found to be most effective in reducing patient symptoms, although conjugated estrogens produced the most cytologic change and the greatest increase in serum levels of estradiol and estrone.

Finally, the effect of different dosages was examined. Low-dose vaginal estradiol was found to be the most efficacious according to symptom relief, although oral estriol was also effective. Estriol had no effect on the serum levels of estradiol or estrone, whereas vaginal estriol had minimal effect. Vaginal estradiol was found to have a small effect on serum estrogen, although not as great as systemic preparations. In conclusion, it would appear that estrogen is efficacious in the treatment of urogenital atrophy, and low-dose vaginal preparations are as effective as systemic therapy.

More recently, the use of a continuous low-dose estradiol-releasing silicone vaginal ring (Estring; Pharmacia and Upjohn, Sweden), releasing estradiol 5–10 μg over 24 hours, has been investigated in postmenopausal women with symptomatic urogenital atrophy.[74] There was a significant effect on symptoms of vaginal dryness, pruritus vulvae, dyspareunia, and urinary urgency, with improvement being reported in over 90% of women in an uncontrolled study. The patient acceptability was high and while the maturation of vaginal epithelium (Figure 5.10) was significantly improved, there was no effect on endometrial proliferation.

Conclusions

Estrogens are known to have an important physiologic effect on the female lower genital tract throughout adult life, leading to symptomatic, histologic, and functional changes. Urogenital atrophy is the manifestation of estrogen withdrawal following the menopause, presenting with vaginal and/or urinary symptoms. The use of estrogen replacement therapy has been examined in the management of lower urinary tract symptoms as well as in the treatment of urogenital atrophy, although only recently has it been subjected to randomized placebo-controlled trials and meta-analysis.

Whereas estrogen therapy alone has been shown to have little effect in the management of urodynamic stress incontinence, when considering the irritative symptoms of urinary urgency, frequency, and urge incontinence, estrogen therapy may be of benefit. However, this may simply represent reversal of urogenital atrophy rather than a direct effect on the lower urinary tract. The role of estrogen replacement therapy in the management of women with recurrent lower urinary tract infection remains to be determined, although

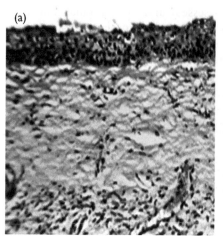
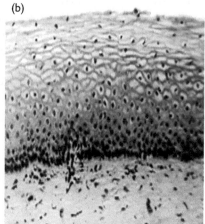

Figure 5.10 Topical vaginal estrogen replacement increases the number of intermediate and superficial cells in the vaginal mucosa: (a) prior to treatment and (b) following treatment. (See also color image on p. xxiii)

there is now some evidence that vaginal administration may be efficacious. Finally, low-dose vaginal estrogens have been shown to have a role in the treatment of urogenital atrophy in postmenopausal women and would appear to be as effective as systemic preparations.

References

1. Cardozo LD. Role of estrogens in the treatment of female urinary incontinence. J Am Geriatr Soc 1990;38:326–8.
2. Iosif CS, Batra S, Ek A, Astedt B. Estrogen receptors in the human female lower urinary tract. Am J Obstet Gynecol 1981;141:817–20.
3. Batra SC, Fossil CS. Female urethra, a target for estrogen action. J Urol 1983;129:418–20.
4. Batra SC, Iosif CS. Progesterone receptors in the female urinary tract. J Urol 1987;138:1301–4.
5. Iosif CS, Bekassy Z. Prevalence of genito-urinary symptoms in the late menopause. Acta Obstet Gynecol Scand 1984;63:257–60.
6. Green S, Walter P, Kumar V, et al. Human estrogen receptor cDNA: sequence, expression and homology to v-erbA. Nature 1986;320:134–9.
7. Kuiper G, Enmark E, Pelto-Huikko M, Nilsson S, Gustafsson J-A. Cloning of a novel estrogen receptor expressed in rat prostate and ovary. Proc Natl Acad Sci USA 1996;93:5925–30.
8. Blakeman PJ, Hilton P, Bulmer JN. Mapping estrogen and progesterone receptors throughout the female lower urinary tract. Neurourol Urodyn 1996; 15:324–5.

9. Ingelman-Sundberg A, Rosen J, Gustafsson SA. Cytosol estrogen receptors in urogenital tissues in stress incontinent women. Acta Obstet Gynecol Scand 1981;60:585–6.

10. Smith P. Estrogens and the urogenital tract. Acta Obstet Gynecol Scand 1993;72:1–26.

11. Bernstein IT. The pelvic floor muscles: muscle thickness in healthy and urinary-incontinent women measured by perineal ultrasonography with reference to the effect of pelvic floor training. Estrogen receptor studies. Neurourol Urodyn 1997;16(4):237–75.

12. Chen GD, Oliver RH, Leung BS, Lin LY, Yeh J. Estrogen receptor α and β expression in the vaginal walls and uterosacral ligaments of premenopausal and postmenopausal women. Fertil Steril 1999;71(6):1099–102.

13. Screiter F, Fuchs P, Stockamp K. Estrogenic sensitivity of α receptors in the urethral musculature. Urol Int 1976;31:13–19.

14. Pang X, Cotreau-Bibbo MM, Sant GR, Theoharides TC. Bladder mast cell expression of high affinity oestrogen receptors in patients with interstitial cystitis. Br J Urol 1995;75:154–61.

15. Rud T, Anderson KE, Asmussen M, et al. Factors maintaining the urethral pressure in women. Invest Urol 1980;17:343–7.

16. Malone-Lee J. Urodynamic measurement and urinary incontinence in the elderly. In: Brocklehurst JC, ed. Managing and measuring incontinence. Proceedings of the Geriatric Workshop on Incontinence, July 1988.

17. Versi E, Cardozo LD. Estrogens and lower urinary tract function. In: Studd JWW, Whitehead MI, eds. The Menopause. Oxford: Blackwell Scientific Publications;1988:76–84.

18. Kinn AC, Lindskog M. Estrogens and phenylpropanolamine in combination for stress incontinence. Urology 1988;32:273–80.

19. Shapiro E. Effect of estrogens on the weight and muscarinic receptor density of the rabbit bladder and urethra. J Urol 1986;135:1084–7.

20. Batra S, Andersson KE. Oestrogen-induced changes in muscarinic receptor density and contractile responses in the female rabbit urinary bladder. Acta Physiol Scand 1989;137:135–41.

21. Elliott RA, Castleden CM, Miodrag A, Kirwan P. The direct effects of diethyl-stilboestrol and nifedipine on the contractile responses of isolated human and rat detrusor muscles. Eur J Clin Pharmacol 1992;43:149–55.

22. Shenfield OZ, Blackmore PF, Morgan CW, et al. Rapid effects of oestriol and progesterone on tone and spontaneous rhythmic contractions of the rabbit bladder. Neurourol Urodyn 1998;17(4):408–9.

23. Fantl JA, Wyman JF, Anderson RL, et al. Postmenopausal urinary incontinence: comparison between non-estrogen-supplemented and estrogen-supplemented women. Obstet Gynecol 1988;71:823–8.

24. Maggi A, Perez J. Role of female gonadal hormones in the CNS. Life Sci 1985;37:893–906.

25. Smith SS, Berg G, Hammar M, eds. The modern management of the menopause. Hormones, mood and neurobiology – a summary. Carnforth, UK: Parthenon Publishing;1993:204.

26. Bergman A, Karram MM, Bhatia NN. Changes in urethral cytology following estrogen administration. Gynaecol Obstet Invest 1990;29:211–13.

27. Rud T. The effects of estrogens and gestagens on the urethral pressure profile in urinary continent and stress incontinent women. Acta Obstet Gynecol Scand 1980;59:265–70.

28. Hilton P, Stanton SL. The use of intravaginal estrogen cream in genuine stress incontinence. Br J Obstet Gynaecol 1983;90:940–4.

29. Bhatia NN, Bergman A, Karram MM, et al. Effects of estrogen on urethral function in women with urinary incontinence. Am J Obstet Gynecol 1989;160:176–80.

30. Karram MM, Yeko TR, Sauer MV, Bhatia NN. Urodynamic changes following hormonal replacement therapy in women with premature ovarian failure. Obstet Gynecol 1989;74:208–11.

31. Versi E, Cardozo LD. Urethral instability: diagnosis based on variations in the maximum urethral pressure in normal climateric women. Neurourol Urodyn 1986;5:535–41.

32. Falconer C, Ekman-Ordeberg G, Ulmsten U, et al. Changes in paraurethral connective tissue at menopause are counteracted by estrogen. Maturitas 1996;24:197–204.

33. Kushner L, Chen Y, Desautel M, et al. Collagenase activity is elevated in conditioned media from fibroblasts of women with pelvic floor weakening. Int Urogynaecol 1999;10(S1):34.

34. Jackson S, Avery N, Shepherd A, et al. The effect of estradiol on vaginal collagen in postmenopausal women with stress urinary incontinence. Nurourol Urodyn 1996;15:327–8.

35. James M, Avery N, Jackson S, Bailey A, Abrams P. The pathophysiological changes of vaginal skin tissue in women with stress urinary incontinence: a controlled trial. Int Urogynaecol 1999;10(S1):35.

36. James M, Avery N, Jackson S, Bailey A, Abrams P. The biochemical profile of vaginal tissue in women with genitourinary prolapse: a controlled trial. Neurourol Urodyn 1999;18(4):284–5.

37. Samsioe G. Urogenital aging – a hidden problem. Am J Obstet Gynecol 1998;178(5):S245–9.

38. Bachman GA. Urogenital aging: an old problem newly recognised. Maturitas 1995;22:S1–5.

39. Kondo A, Kato K, Saito M, et al. Prevalence of hand washing incontinence in females in comparison with stress and urge incontinence. Neurourol Urodyn 1990;9:330–1.

40. Thomas TM, Plymat KR, Blannin J, Meade TW. Prevalence of urinary incontinence. Br Med J 1980;281:1243–5.

41. Jolleys JV. Reported prevalence of urinary incontinence in a general practice. Br Med J 1988;296:1300–2.

42. Burgio KL, Matthews KA, Engel B. Prevalence, incidence and correlates of urinary incontinence in healthy, middle-aged women. J Urol 1991;146:1255–9.

43. Sandford JP. Urinary tract symptoms and infection. Ann Rev Med 1975;26:485–505.

44. Boscia JA, Kaye D. Assymptomatic bacteria in the elderly. Infect Dis Clin North Am 1987;1:893–903.

45. Salmon UL, Walter RI, Gast SH. The use of estrogen in the treatment of dysuria and incontinence in postmenopausal women. Am J Obstet Gynecol 1941; 14:23–31.

46. Youngblood VH, Tomlin EM, Davis JB. Senile urethritis in women. J Urol 1957;78:150–2.

47. Fantl JA, Cardozo LD, McClish DK and the Hormones and Urogenital Therapy Committee. Estrogen therapy in the management of incontinence in postmenopausal women: a meta-analysis. First report of the Hormones and Urogenital Therapy Committee. Obstet Gynecol 1994;83:12–18.

48. Henalla SM, Hutchins CJ, Robinson P, Macivar J. Non-operative methods in the treatment of female genuine stress incontinence of urine. Br J Obstet Gynaecol 1989;9:222–5.

49. Zullo MA, Oliva C, Falconi G, Paparella P, Mancuso S. Efficacy of estrogen therapy in urinary incontinence. A meta-analytic study. Minerva Ginecol 1998;50(5):199–205.

50. Grady D, Brown JS, Vittinghoff E, et al. Postmenopausal hormones and incontinence: the Heart and Estrogen/Progestin Replacement Study. Obstet Gynecol 2001;97:116–20.

51. Grodstein F, Lifford K, Resnick NM, Curhan GC. Postmenopausal hormone therapy and risk of developing urinary incontinence. Obstet Gynecol 2004;103:254–60.

52. Ouslander JG, Greendale GA, et al. Effects of oral estrogen and progestin on the lower urinary tract among female nursing home residents. Am Geriatr Soc 2001;49(6):803–7.

53. Moehrer B, Hextall A, Jackson S. Oestrogens for urinary incontinence in women. Cochrane Database Syst Rev 2003;(2):CD001405.

54. Caine M, Raz S. The role of female hormones in stress incontinence. In: Proceedings of the 16th Congress of the International Society of Urology, Amsterdam, the Netherlands.

55. Rud T. The effects of estrogens and gestagens on the urethral pressure profile in urinary continent and stress incontinent women. Acta Obstet Gynecol Scand 1980;59:265–70.

56. Wilson PD, Faragher B, Butler B, et al. Treatment with oral piperazine oestrone sulphate for genuine stress incontinence in postmenopausal women. Br J Obstet Gynaecol 1987;94:568–74.

57. Walter S, Wolf H, Barlebo H, Jansen H. Urinary incontinence in postmenopausal women treated with estrogens: a double-blind clinical trial. J Urol 1978;33:135–43.

58. Fantl JA, Bump RC, Robinson D, et al. Efficacy of estrogen supplementation in the treatment of urinary incontinence. Obstet Gynecol 1996;88:745–9.

59. Jackson S, Shepherd A, Brookes S, Abrams P. The effect of estrogen supplementation on post-menopausal urinary stress incontinence: a double-blind, placebo controlled trial. Br J Obstet Gynaecol 1999;106:711–18.

60. Sultana CJ, Walters MD. Estrogen and urinary incontinence in women. Maturitas 1995;20:129–38.

61. Al-Badr A, Ross S, Soroka D, Drutz HP. What is the available evidence for hormone replacement therapy in women with stress urinary incontinence? J Obstet Gynaecol Can 2003;25(7):567–74.

62. Samsioe G, Jansson I, Mellstrom D, Svanborg A. Urinary incontinence in 75-year-old women. Effects of oestriol. Acta Obstet Gynecol Scand 1985;93:57.

63. Cardozo LD, Rekers H, Tapp A, et al. Oestriol in the treatment of post-menopausal urgency: a multicentre study. Maturitas 1993;18:47–53.
64. Benness C, Wise BG, Cutner A, Cardozo LD. Does low dose vaginal estradiol improve frequency and urgency in postmenopausal women? Int Urogynaecol J 1992;3(2):281.
65. Eriksen PS, Rasmussen H. Low-dose 17β-estradiol vaginal tablets in the treatment of atrophic vaginitis: a double-blind placebo controlled study. Eur J Obstet Gynecol Reprod Biol 1992;44:137–44.
66. Hendrix SL, Cochrane BB, Nygaard, IE, et al. Effects of estrogen with and without progestin on urinary incontinence. JAMA 2005;293(8):935–48.
67. Brandberg A, Mellstrom D, Samsioe G. Low dose oral oestriol treatment in elderly women with urogenital infections. Acta Obstet Gynecol Scand Suppl 1987;140:33–8.
68. Parsons CL, Schmidt JD. Control of recurrent urinary tract infections in postmenopausal women. J Urol 1982;128:1224–6.
69. Privette M, Cade R, Peterson J, et al. Prevention of recurrent urinary tract infections in postmenopausal women. Nephron 1988;50:24–7.
70. Kjaergaard B, Walter S, Knudsen A, Johansen B, Barlebo H. [Treatment with low-dose vaginal estradiol in postmenopausal women. A double-blind controlled trial]. Ugeskr Laeger 1990;152:658–9. [Danish]
71. Raz R, Stamm WE. A controlled trial of intravaginal oestriol in postmenopausal women with recurrent urinary tract infections. N Engl J Med 1993;329:753–6.
72. Kirkengen AL, Andersen P, Gjersoe E, et al. Oestriol in the prophylactic treatment of recurrent urinary tract infections in postmenopausal women. Scand J Prim Health Care 1992;10:139–42.
73. Cardozo LD, Benness C, Abbott D. Low dose estrogen prophylaxis for recurrent urinary tract infections in elderly women. Br J Obstet Gynaecol 1998;105:403–7.
74. Eriksen B. A randomized, open, parallel-group study on the preventive effect of an estradiol-releasing vaginal ring (Estring) on recurrent urinary tract infections in postmenopausal women. Am J Obstet Gynaecol 1999;180:1072–9.
75. Mettler L, Olsen PG. Long-term treatment of atrophic vaginitis with low-dose estradiol vaginal tablets. Maturitas 1991;14:23–31.
76. Smith P, Heimer G, Lindskog, Ulmsten U. Oestradiol-releasing vaginal ring for treatment of postmenopausal urogenital atrophy. Maturitas 1993;16:145–54.
77. Smith RJN, Studd JWW. Recent advances in hormone replacement therapy. Br J Hosp Med 1993;49:799–809.
78. Cardozo LD, Bachmann G, McClish D, Fonda D, Birgerson L. Meta-analysis of estrogen therapy in the management of urogenital atrophy in postmenopausal women: second report of the Hormones and Urogenital Therapy Committee. Obstet Gynecol 1998;92:722–7.

Chapter 6

Diagnosis and evaluation of urinary incontinence and pelvic organ prolapse

Sujatha Rajan and Neeraj Kohli

Introduction

Based on data from the Bureau of Census, postmenopausal women will comprise 33% of the population in the year 2050 compared with 23% in 1995. Since incontinence and pelvic organ prolapse (POP) predominantly affect perimenopausal and postmenopausal women, the numbers of women affected with these conditions, as well as the demand for evaluation and treatment, is projected to steadily increase.

Urinary incontinence (UI), or the unintentional loss of urine, is a problem for more than 13 million Americans, 85% of them women.[1,2] Despite its widespread prevalence, UI is widely underdiagnosed and underreported. For POP, the prevalence varies from 7 to 25%, with a woman's lifetime risk of needing surgery for POP being reported as 11% by age 80. In this chapter, we will confine ourselves to the diagnosis and evaluation of urinary incontinence initially, and then discuss pelvic organ prolapse.

Types of urinary incontinence

The five most common subtypes of urinary incontinence are stress incontinence, urge incontinence, mixed incontinence, overflow incontinence, and functional incontinence. *Stress incontinence* is defined as an involuntary loss of urine with any increase in intra-abdominal pressure (coughing, laughing, sneezing, etc). It is commonly attributed to either loss of urethrovesical supports, i.e. urethral hypermobility, or a deficient urethral sphincter mechanism. *Urge incontinence* (overactive bladder) is defined as the involuntary loss of urine associated with an urge to void. It is caused by uninhibited detrusor contractions and is often accompanied by urinary frequency and nocturia. Women who have both genuine stress incontinence and overactive bladder are said to have *mixed incontinence*. For these patients, it is helpful to identify the most bothersome symptom and treat accordingly. *Overflow incontinence* is the involuntary loss of urine associated with incomplete bladder emptying. This type of incontinence may have a variety of presentations, including urinary frequency, constant dribbling, and urge or stress incontinence symptoms. Overflow UI is either due to an underactive or acontractile detrusor muscle, or due to bladder outlet obstruction. It is important to recognize this condition early to prevent hydronephrosis and renal damage if ureteral reflux were to occur. Overflow incontinence is more common in men and is usually secondary to obstructive prostatic hypertrophy. *Functional incontinence* is leakage of urine due to the inability of the patient to reach the toilet on time. It is usually associated with chronic impairment of physical or cognitive functioning. *Anatomic incontinence* can be congenital (i.e. ectopic ureter) or iatrogenic (i.e. postsurgical or post radiation fistula).

Initial assessment of urinary incontinence

Purpose

The purpose of the initial assessment is to:[3]

- establish a presumptive condition-specific diagnosis and exclude other organ-specific conditions that require intervention
- assess the level of bother and the desire for intervention
- institute disease-specific therapy
- identify patients who require further complex testing or specialist referral.

Components

Components of the initial assessment include obtaining a history, physical examination, measurement of post-void residual volume, and urinalysis (Figure 6.1).

History

Patients with urinary incontinence have typically endured this condition for a long period of time and are often embarrassed to discuss it. Valuable information that could otherwise be missed during a verbal history-taking can be obtained by having patients fill out a structured questionnaire (Table 6.1). These instruments should focus on assessing the type and severity of incontinence as well as its impact on the patient's life. Risk factors that are associated with UI and POP should be identified and attempts must be made to modify them. Table 6.2 lists the reversible causes of urinary incontinence and their management. The medical history should also identify such contributing factors as diabetes, stroke, lumbar disk disease, chronic lung disease, fecal impaction, heart disease, glaucoma, obesity, and cognitive impairment. The obstetric and gynecologic history should include

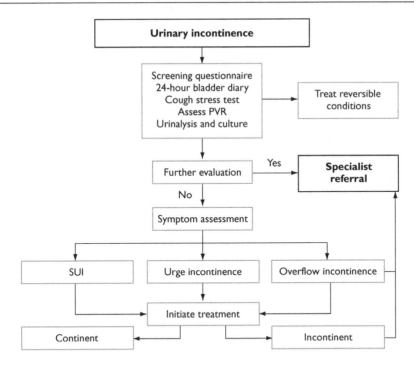

Figure 6.1 Evaluation and management algorithm for urinary incontinence. PVR = post-void residual, SUI = stress urinary incontinence.

gravidity, parity, number of vaginal deliveries, instrument-assisted and cesarean deliveries, pelvic surgeries (hysterectomy, incontinence procedures, and reconstructive surgery), pelvic radiotherapy, trauma, and estrogen status.

Information on the patient's profession/lifestyle, with specific inquiry regarding chronic heavy lifting, nature of exercise, sexual activity, tobacco use, daily fluid, caffeine, and alcohol intake, are also useful. A complete list of all medications that the patient consumes is also essential. Antipsychotics, anticholinergics, sedative hypnotics, calcium channel blockers, α-adrenergic agonists, and other blockers and diuretics are some of the commonly used medications that could cause urinary incontinence.

Bladder diaries are helpful supplements to history-taking in many patients.[4-6] These written records kept over a 24–48-hour period are helpful in determining urinary frequency, functional bladder capacity, and fluid intake as well as other factors associated with UI. These records also provide clues about the underlying cause/nature of UI, and are often helpful in patient education and to instigate behavioral modification. They also serve as a baseline to assess severity and treatment efficacy. A recent report by Williams concluded that a large proportion of women with urodynamic stress incontinence can be accurately diagnosed by clinical history alone

Table 6.1 Sample questionnaire for the evaluation of urinary incontinence and prolapse

How long have you leaked urine?

Do you wear protection for incontinence? How many pads per day?

How many times do you urinate in a 24-hour period?

How many times do you wake up to urinate (each night)?

Do you ever feel a strong sense of urgency to urinate?

Do you ever leak urine after a strong sense of urgency?

Do you have pain or burning when you urinate?

Is your urine ever bloody?

Do you lose urine accidentally with laughing, sneezing, exercising, coughing, lifting, or standing up?

Do you find you've had leakage without being aware?

Do you feel that your bladder empties completely?

Do you ever strain or push to urinate?

Do you dribble urine after urinating?

Do you have to lean over or stand to urinate?

Do you wait a long time before the urine comes out?

Do you have a sense of your pelvic organs 'falling out'?

Do you notice anything protruding from the vagina?

Do you have difficulty with your bowel movements?

Do you have to splint the vagina or perineum to evacuate your bowels or bladder?

Are you incontinent of stool?

(sensitivity 0.92; specificity 0.56). Williams et al[7] have reported that the urinary diary was the most cost-effective test to aid in the diagnosis in a primary care setting.

Physical examination

Physical examination should focus on the following:

- The level of alertness and functional status.
- Documentation of height and weight, since an elevated body mass index is one of the risk factors for UI.
- Evidence of fluid overload, especially in patients with urinary frequency and nocturia.
- Presence of intra-abdominal or pelvic masses and tenderness.

Table 6.2 Transient (reversible) conditions that cause or contribute to urinary incontinence

Condition or finding	Management
Detectable by history	
Drug side-effects	Discontinue or change medication, if possible
Delirium or hypoxia	Treat underlying cause
Recent prostatectomy	Behavioral therapy
Excessive fluid intake	Reduction of fluid intake
Impaired mobility	Physical therapy or environmental changes (bedside commode)
Detectable by physical examination	
Atrophic vaginitis	Estrogen therapy
Fecal impaction	Disimpaction and stool softeners
Venous insufficiency and edema	Leg elevation, stockings, sodium restriction
Detectable by urinalysis	
Urinary tract infection	Antibiotic therapy
Glycosuria	Control diabetes

- A neurological examination to rule out multiple sclerosis and spinal cord compression. Specific emphasis should be placed on assessing the sacral nerve roots. This includes checking: deep tendon reflexes at the knee and ankle; lower extremity strength, abduction and dorsiflexion at the toes (S3); sensory innervation of the labia minora (L1–L2); sole and lateral aspect of the foot (S1); posterior aspect of thigh (S2); perineum (S3); and the bulbocavernosus and clitoral sacral reflexes (Figure 6.2). Abnormal findings such as deep tendon hyperreflexia or absence of the bulbocavernosus reflex should alert the physician to possible underlying neurologic lesions contributing to urinary incontinence.
- Pelvic examination should look for evidence of vaginal atrophy. The most common signs of inadequate estrogen levels are thinning and paleness of the vaginal epithelium, loss of rugae, disappearance of the labia minora, and presence of a urethral caruncle. A *urethral diverticulum* usually presents as a mass on the distal anterior vaginal wall. Gentle massage of this mass may produce a purulent discharge from the urethral meatus.
- A bimanual examination is performed to assess the size, shape, and position of the uterus. A large uterus directly over the bladder or incarcerated in the pelvis could cause or exacerbate urinary urgency, frequency, stress incontinence, and at times could cause bladder outlet obstruction.

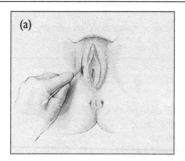 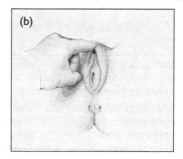

Figure 6.2 (a) Bulbocavernosus and (b) clitoral sacral reflexes. Lightly tapping the clitoris or brushing the labia majora should produce a reflex contraction of the external anal sphincter muscle. Reproduced with permission from Culligan PJ, Heit M. Urinary incontinence in women: evaluation and management. Am Fam Physician 2000;62(11): 2433–44. (See also color image on p. xxiii)

- While performing the bimanual examination, levator ani muscle function can be evaluated by asking the patient to tighten around a finger placed in the vagina and to hold the contraction as long as possible. Very weak or absent voluntary levator ani muscle contractions are an indication that biofeedback training sessions with a pelvic floor physical therapist may be helpful.
- A rectal examination is then done to check anal sphincter tone and to look for fecal impaction and the presence of occult blood or rectal lesions.
- In all women with UI a detailed examination should be done to identify associated pelvic organ prolapse. This examination is described in detail later in this chapter.

Q TIP TEST

This is a test designed to assess urethral hypermobility, and it can be done by either a visual examination, with a Q tip, which is the commonly employed technique, by ultrasound, bead chain cystourethrography, or videocystourethrography. To perform this test, the patient is placed in the dorsal lithotomy position, and hypermobility is measured by placing a lubricated, sterile, cotton-tipped applicator into the urethra at the level of the urethrovesical junction. The resting angle is documented and then the patient is asked to strain down. This allows the tail of the applicator to transcribe an arc, which is then measured with a goniometer. Urethral hypermobility is defined by a maximal strain axis greater than $+30°$. This test does not distinguish women with stress incontinence from continent subjects and these days is used primarily to evaluate the results of incontinence surgery or to determine whether the degree of urethral hypermobility may influence surgical outcomes.[8]

Estimation of post-void residual (PVR) volume

As part of the basic evaluation, the PVR volume should be estimated in all patients to diagnose urinary retention. Prior to starting the examination, the patient is asked to void and the amount is measured. The PVR volume is then measured either by catheterization or with an ultrasound. In general, PVR volumes of less than 50 ml are considered adequate bladder emptying. Repetitive PVR volumes over 100 ml are considered inadequate emptying and require further evaluation, including urodynamic testing.[2] Measurements made using a portable ultrasound have been found to be 84–95% accurate.[9,10]

Urinalysis

Urinalysis is used to detect conditions that are associated with or contributing to UI, such as hematuria (suggestive of infection, cancer or stone), glycosuria (which may cause polyuria and contribute to UI symptoms), pyuria and bacteriuria, as well as proteinuria. If catheterization is performed for PVR volume measurement, a sample of the residual urine can be used for the urinalysis and microscopic examination. The value of urinalysis in the evaluation of urinary incontinence is illustrated by the fact that 60% of women with a stable bladder will develop detrusor overactivity during a urinary tract infection. The clinical relevance of asymptomatic bacteriuria without pyuria and vice versa is controversial and many suggest treatment of either condition.[11,12]

Office tests for the evaluation of urinary incontinence

Cough stress test

After filling the bladder to 300 ml using a catheter, the patient is asked to cough once vigorously after the catheter is removed. The urethral meatus is observed for leakage of urine. If an instantaneous leakage occurs with cough, then stress urinary incontinence (SUI) is likely; if leakage is delayed or persists after the cough, detrusor overactivity should be suspected. The test is initially performed in the lithotomy position and, if leakage is not observed, it should be repeated in the upright position. Often a series of coughs is required to demonstrate incontinence. Women who demonstrate urine leakage in the supine position with a relatively empty bladder (immediately after voiding and confirmation of adequate bladder emptying) are at increased risk of having intrinsic sphincter deficiency.[13]

In women with significant pelvic organ prolapse, testing for potential SUI is advocated. Potential incontinence is occult incontinence, which is manifested only upon reduction of the prolapse. In these women, incontinence remains occult as a result of kinking of the urethra while the prolapse protrudes through the vagina. To unmask this condition, the prolapse is reduced either manually, or with a pessary or large cotton swabs, and a cough stress test is performed as described earlier. Studies have shown that, with the prolapse reduced, incontinence can occur in 30–50% of patients with advanced prolapse.

Pad test

The objective of this test is to document the volume of urine loss using a perineal pad, before and after some type of leakage provocation. A 1-hour pad test is typically conducted. Generally, the test begins with the woman emptying her bladder and then drinking a known amount of water, typically 500 ml. Alternatively, the bladder can be filled with a set amount or to maximum capacity. The pad is weighed after 1 hour of activity for a short-term pad test conducted in the office, or after 24–48 hours during the long-term pad test conducted at home. A pad weight gain of >1 g during 1 hour, or >4 g during 24 hours is considered positive. Controversy exists regarding the reproducibility and validity of these tests.[14,15] A specific use for the pad test is when the clinician is unsure if the symptoms of incontinence are a result of urine loss or secondary to vaginal secretions or sweating. By giving the woman phenazopyridine hydrochloride (Pyridium) to turn her urine orange, a pad test can confirm urine loss.

Urodynamic testing

These specialized tests are indicated in patients with mixed incontinence, complex or unclear etiology of UI, recurrent incontinence, neurogenic bladder, or a history of previous pelvic surgery. Urodynamic testing is discussed in Chapter 8.

Other tests

Blood testing – blood urea nitrogen (BUN), creatinine, glucose, and calcium – is recommended if compromised renal function is suspected or if polyuria (in the absence of diuretics) is present. Urine cytology is not recommended in the routine evaluation of the incontinent patient.

Diagnostic evaluation in patients with prolapse

Most elements of the history are similar to those described earlier in the section on urinary incontinence (see Table 6.1). Symptoms of prolapse are not specific to different compartments but may reflect the overall stage of prolapse at its most advanced site. Women may find that they are unable to wear tampons and often complain of a sense of pressure and heaviness. A palpable bulge is usually reported after the prolapse extends beyond the genital hiatus. Although back pain has been considered a classic symptom of prolapse, a recent study has shown that women with more advanced prolapse actually had less back pain than women with mild prolapse.[16] Women with prolapse often have urinary symptoms, including urgency, incontinence, or symptoms of urethral obstruction (hesitancy, frequency, and incomplete emptying). In one study, urethral obstruction occurred in 58% of women with grade 3 and 4 anterior vaginal prolapse, compared with 4% in women with grade 1 and 2 prolapse.[17] As prolapse advances, women are less likely to have stress incontinence and more likely to manually reduce prolapse to void. Defecatory symptoms such as excessive straining, incomplete rectal emptying, or the need for perineal or vaginal pressure to accomplish defecation should be sought in all women with prolapse. In addition, the influence of prolapse on sexual functioning should be addressed in women of all ages.[18]

Traditionally, assessments of POP were performed in the supine position. However, the pelvic supports that hold the pelvic organs in place were designed to function in the standing position; this is the orientation in which the pelvic organ supports must be evaluated. A site-specific assessment of pelvic floor defects is recommended in the lithotomy position as well as with the patient standing. It is crucial to have the patient maximally straining while these measurements are being taken. All measurements are made using the hymen as the reference mark. Initially, a double-bladed speculum is used to assess the cervix or the vaginal apex. The blades of the speculum are then separated and the posterior blade is used to depress the posterior vaginal wall while assessing defects in the anterior compartment. The blade is removed and repositioned to retract the anterior vaginal wall while assessing the posterior compartment. Special attention should be given to the size of the genital hiatus, since women with larger genital openings could have difficulty retaining a pessary.

Historically, prolapse was graded using a variety of classification systems that were not easily reproduced or communicated in a standard way among clinicians. The older classification systems included the Baden and Walker[19] halfway system and the revised New York Classification (NYC) system. Since its introduction in 1996 and adoption by the Society of Gynecologic Surgeons, American Urogynecologic Society, and International Continence Society, the Pelvic Organ Prolapse Quantification (POP-Q) system has become the most common standardized grading system used in the medical literature.[20] It has proven inter- and intraobserver reliability.[21] This grading system involves quantitative measurements of various points representing anterior, apical, posterior, and basal vaginal prolapse to create a '9 point topographic' map of the vagina. The fixed point of reference for all POP-Q measurements is the hymen. These anatomic points can then be used to determine the stage of the prolapse.

Measurements

Two points are located on the anterior vaginal wall:

• Point Aa is located at the midline of the anterior vaginal wall, 3 cm proximal to the external urethral meatus. It corresponds approximately to the urethrovesical junction and may be located anywhere from −3 to +3 cm from the hymen, depending upon the extent of anterior wall prolapse.
• Point Ba is the most distal position of any part of the upper anterior vaginal wall from the vaginal cuff or anterior vaginal fornix to point Aa.

Two points are located in the superior vagina:

• Point C is the most distal (i.e. most dependent) edge of the cervix or the leading edge of the vaginal cuff after hysterectomy.
• Point D is the deepest point of the posterior fornix in a woman who still has a cervix. It is usually located where the uterosacral ligaments attach to the posterior cervix. Measuring this point distinguishes between suspensory failure of the uterosacral-cardinal ligament complex and cervical elongation: if point C is significantly more positive than point D (e.g. greater than 4 cm), the cervix is elongated.

Two points are measured on the posterior vaginal wall, analogous to the two points on the anterior wall:

• Point Ap is located in the midline of the posterior vaginal wall, 3 cm proximal to the hymen. This point ranges from −3 in a normal woman to +3 when there is complete vaginal prolapse.
• Point Bp is the most distal (i.e. most dependent) position of any part of the upper posterior vaginal wall from the vaginal cuff or posterior vaginal fornix to point Ap.

Three additional measurements are:

• The genital hiatus (GH) is measured from the middle of the external urethral meatus to the posterior midline hymen. If the location of the hymen is obscured by a band of skin (usually from surgery or episiotomy repair), the firm tissue of the perineal body is the posterior margin of this measurement.

- The perineal body (PB) is measured from the posterior margin of the genital hiatus to the midanal opening.
- The total vaginal length (TVL) is measured as the greatest depth of the vagina when point C or D is reduced completely to its normal position.

All measurements are expressed in centimeters and can be marked on line diagrams or a tic-tac-toe grid (Figure 6.3) or recorded individually.

There are five stages of pelvic organ support (0 through IV) as follows:

- Stage 0: no prolapse is demonstrated.
- Stage I: the criteria for stage 0 are not met, but the most distal portion of the prolapse is >1 cm above the level of the hymen.
- Stage II: the most distal portion of the prolapse is ≤1 cm proximal to or distal to the plane of the hymen (i.e. its quantitation value ≥−1 cm but ≤+1 cm).
- Stage III: the most distal portion of the prolapse is >1 cm below the plane of the hymen but protrudes no further than 2 cm less than the total vaginal length in centimeters (i.e. its quantitation value is >+1 cm but <+[TVL−2] cm).

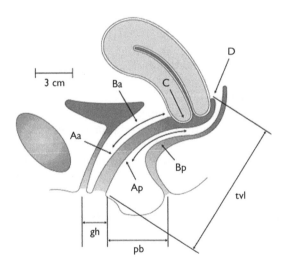

Figure 6.3 Diagram representation of the pelvic organ prolapse quantitation system for staging prolapse by physical examination findings, showing the 6 sites (points Aa and Ba anteriorly, points Ap and Bp posteriorly, point C for the cervix or apex, and point D for the cul-de-sac), genital hiatus (gh), perineal body (pb), and total vaginal length (tvl) used for pelvic organ prolapse quantitation. (Reproduced with permission from Weber and Richter.[22])

- Stage IV: essentially, complete eversion of the total length of the vagina. The distal portion of the prolapse protrudes to at least (TVL−2) cm (i.e. its quantitation value is greater or equal to +[TVL−2] cm).

Pelvic floor muscle function should be assessed in all women.[23] The levators can be palpated at 4 and 8 o'clock positions a few centimeters internal to the hymen. The resting and squeeze tone, and the strength, duration, and symmetry of the squeeze should be recorded. Women who are unable to generate an adequate squeeze may benefit from supervised instruction and physical therapy.

Supplemental physical examination techniques for evaluating prolapse

These techniques are essential for adequate assessment of prolapse and may be helpful in preoperative planning. They include:

1. Digital rectovaginal examination while the patient is straining to differentiate between a high rectocele and an enterocele.
2. Digital assessment of the contents of the rectovaginal septum to differentiate between a 'traction' enterocele (the posterior cul-de-sac is pulled down with the prolapsing cervix or vaginal cuff but is not distended by intestines) and a 'pulsion' enterocele (the intestinal contents of the enterocele distend the rectal–vaginal septum and produce a protruding mass).
3. Measurements of perineal descent.
4. Measurements of the transverse diameter of the genital hiatus or of the protruding prolapse.
5. Measurements of vaginal volume.
6. Description and measurement of rectal prolapse.
7. Examination techniques for differentiating between various types of defects: e.g. central (Figure 6.4) vs paravaginal (Figure 6.5) defects of the anterior vaginal wall.

Ancillary tests for pelvic organ prolapse

These POP tests are not routinely recommended but may be helpful in some patients to provide a better understanding of the prolapse.

Endoscopy

Cystoscopy and sigmoidoscopy may play a role in the evaluation of POP. For example, cystoscopic observation of peristalsis under the bladder trigone can identify an anterior enterocele. Sigmoidoscopy may help to

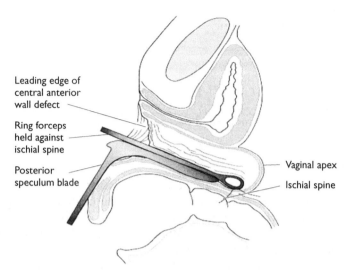

Leading edge of
central anterior
wall defect

Ring forceps
held against
ischial spine

Posterior
speculum blade

Vaginal apex

Ischial spine

Figure 6.4 The examiner checks for a central defect by inserting the posterior speculum blade, placing the tips of an opened ring forceps against the lateral vaginal wall (one against each ischial spine), and asking the patient to strain. If the anterior wall descends, a central defect is present. (Reproduced with permission from Julian.[24])

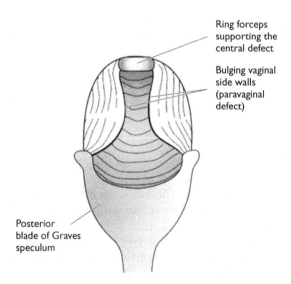

Ring forceps
supporting the
central defect

Bulging vaginal
side walls
(paravaginal
defect)

Posterior
blade of Graves
speculum

Figure 6.5 The examiner checks for a paravaginal defect by placing the shaft of the closed ring forceps directly under the vertical midline of the anterior vaginal wall and asking the patient to strain. If the anterior vaginal wall descends, a paravaginal defect is present. (Reproduced with permission from Julian.[24])

delineate how much of a posterior vaginal wall prolapse is rectosigmoid as opposed to small intestine.

Photography

If prolapse is stage II or greater, photographs that include a centimeter tape as a frame of reference can help objectively document presurgical findings or serial changes in an individual patient.

Imaging

Although imaging techniques have been used to visualize pelvic floor support defects, the lack of standardization and validation of these modalities limit their usefulness. Ultrasonography allows real-time observation of dynamic events such as bladder neck descent during cough. Lately, three-dimensional ultrasound is being used more commonly to describe pelvic floor anatomy and function and offers advantages due to ease of performance.[25] Contrast radiography illustrates mechanisms of micturition and defecation. Magnetic resonance imaging (MRI) is a promising research tool for studying pelvic floor anatomy and pathophysiology.[26]

Pelvic floor muscle testing

Instrumental testing may be performed, but none of these techniques has proven clinical applicability in the assessment of POP. Electromyography with needle electrodes permits visualization of individual motor unit action potentials; surface electrodes detect the activity of groups of motor units. This evaluation may still be investigational and its clinical utility is unclear at this time.

Summary

- Urinary incontinence and Pelvic organ prolapse are very common and distressing conditions.
- Diagnosis of urinary incontinence requires a systematic approach including history, physical exam, estimation of post void residual, and ruling out urinary tract infection.
- Urodynamic testing is needed in 10% of patients with urinary incontinence and is used more frequently among subspecialists due to the complexity of patients referred to them.
- Evaluating the extent of descent of each compartment of pelvic organ support is critical prior to instituting treatment.
- The POPQ system is being more frequently employed for grading pelvic organ prolapse. This system has good inter and intra observer reliability.

- Women with prolapse may have potential stress urinary incontinence and reduction testing is often necessary to diagnose this.

References

1. National Kidney and Urologic Diseases Advisory Board. Barriers to rehabilitation of persons with end-stage renal disease or chronic urinary incontinence. Workshop summary report. March 7–9, 1994, Bethesda, MD.
2. Fantl JA, Newman DK, Colling J, et al. Urinary incontinence in adults: acute and chronic management. Clinical Practice Guideline No. 2, 1996 update. Rockville, Md. US Department of Health and Human Services, Public Health Service, Agency for Health Care Policy and Research, March 1996. AHCPR publication No. 96–0682.
3. 3rd International Consultation on Incontinence, June 2004, Monte Carlo, Monaco.
4. Diokno AC, Wells TJ, Brink CA. Comparison of self-reported voided volume with cystometric bladder capacity. J Urol 1987;137(4):698–700.
5. Larson G, Victor A. The frequency–volume chart in genuine stress incontinent women. Neurourol Urodyn 1992;1:23–31.
6. Wyman JF, Choi SC, Harkins SW, Wilson Ms, Fantl JA. The urinary diary in evaluation of urinary incontinence in women: a test retest analysis. Obstet Gynecol 1988;71(6 pt 1):812–17.
7. Williams K, Martin J, Abrams K, et al. Systematic review and evaluation of methods of diagnostic assessment for urinary incontinence. International Continence Society (ICS) meeting, 2004.
8. Karram MM, Bhatia NN. The Q-tip test: standardization of the technique and its interpretation in women with urinary incontinence. Obstet Gynecol 1988; 71(6 Pt 1):807–11.
9. Borrie MJ, Campbell K, Arcese ZA, et al. Urinary retention in patients in a geriatric rehabilitation unit: prevalence, risk factors, and validity of bladder scan evaluation. Rehabil Nurs 2001;26(5):187–91.
10. Ding YY, Sahadevan S, Pang WS, Choo PW. Clinical utility of a portable ultrasound scanner in the measurement of residual urine volume. Singapore Med J 1996;37(4):365–8.
11. DuBeau CE, Resnick NM. Evaluation of the causes and severity of geriatric incontinence. A critical appraisal. Urol Clin North Am 1991;18(2):243–56.
12. Ouslander JG, Schapira M, Schnelle JF, Fingold S. Pyuria among chronically incontinent but otherwise asymptomatic nursing home residents. J Am Geriatr Soc 1996;44(4):420–3.
13. Lobel RW, Sand PK. The empty supine stress test as a predictor of intrinsic urethral sphincter dysfunction. Obstet Gynecol 1996;88:128–32.
14. Lose G, Fantl JA, Victor A, et al. Outcome measures for research in adult women with symptoms of lower urinary tract dysfunction. Neurourol Urodyn 1998;17:255–62.
15. Artibani W, Andersen JT, Gajewski J, et al. Imaging and other investigations. In: Abrams P, Cardozo L, Khoury S, Wein A, eds. Incontinence, 2nd edn. Plymouth, MA: Health Publication; 2002:425–77.

16. Heit M, Culligan P, Rosenquist C, Shott S. Is pelvic organ prolapse a cause of pelvic or low back pain? Obstet Gynecol 2002;99:23–8.

17. Romanzi LJ, Chaikin DC, Blaivas JG. The effect of genital prolapse on voiding. J Urol 1999;161:581–6.

18. Handa VL, Harvey L, Cundiff GW, Siddique SA, Kjerulff KH. Sexual function among women with urinary incontinence and pelvic organ prolapse. Am J Obstet Gynecol 2004;191:751–6.

19. Baden WF, Walker T, Lindsey JH. The vaginal profile. Tex Med 1968;64: 56–73.

20. Bump RC, Mattiasson A, Bo K, et al. The standardization of terminology of female pelvic organ prolapse and pelvic floor dysfunction. Am J Obstet Gynecol 1996;175(1):10–17.

21. Hall, AF, Theofrastous, JP, Cundiff, GW, et al. Interobserver and intraobserver reliability of the proposed International Continence Society, Society of Gynecologic Surgeons, and American Urogynecologic Society pelvic organ prolapse classification system. Am J Obstet Gynecol 1996;175:1467.

22. Weber AM, Richter HE. Pelvic organ prolapse. Obstet Gynecol 2005; 106:615–34.

23. Brink CA, Wells TJ, Sampselle CM, Taillie ER, Mayer R. A digital test for pelvic muscle strength in women with urinary incontinence. Nurs Res 1994; 43:352–6.

24. Julian JT. Physical examination and pretreatment testing of the incontinent woman. Clin Obstet Gynecol 1998; 41(3): 663–71.

25. Dietz HP. Ultrasound imaging of the pelvic floor. Part II: three-dimensional or volume imaging. Ultrasound Obstet Gynecol 2004;23(6):615–25.

26. Hodroff MA, Stolpen AH, Denson MA, Bolinger L, Kreder KJ. Dynamic magnetic resonance imaging of the female pelvis: the relationship with the pelvic organ prolapse quantification staging system. J Urol 2002;167:1353–5.

Chapter 7

Colorectal evaluation

Samir Yebara and Eric Weiss

Introduction

The mainstay of any evaluation in medicine, including that of the ano-rectum, is a detailed history and physical examination. Various diagnostic and physiologic tests are available in assisting the surgeon in determining a diagnosis (Figure 7.1).

Most patients with anorectal complaints attribute them to 'hemorrhoids'. Often this diagnosis can be ruled in or ruled out by a detailed history and physical examination. Although most anorectal conditions are benign, may be successfully treated by primary care practitioners, and do not require surgical treatment, a high index of suspicion for colorectal cancer should be maintained, and all patients should be appropriately investigated.

History

The combination of the chief complaint and the history of present illness is usually enough information to diagnose most anorectal disorders. A carefully taken history usually establishes the diagnosis or at least suggests it (Table 7.1).

Bleeding

Rectal bleeding can be a sign of many different problems, with a prevalence of 14–19% in adults.[2] Bright red blood may be seen only on toilet paper or in the toilet bowl after a bowel movement. This is usually from hemor-rhoids or an anal fissure. The distinguishing factor is that an anal fissure causes a painful bowel movement, whereas hemorrhoids do not. Bright red rectal bleeding that drips into the bowl and streaks the stool is usually inter-nal hemorrhoids. Blood on the toilet tissue associated with painful bowel movement is frequently an anal fissure. This can be easily diagnosed by direct visual examination (Table 7.2).

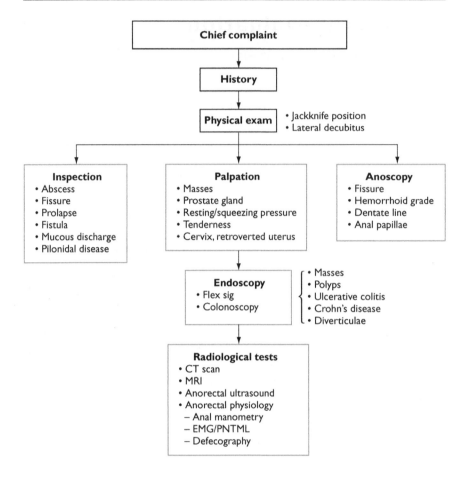

Figure 7.1 Algorithm for colorectal evaluation.

Blood in the stool may also indicate inflammation of colon or rectum such as with inflammatory bowel disease (IBD). Often IBD will present with other symptoms, including diarrhea, cramping, abdominal pain, urgency, and tenesmus. Colitis or proctitis may be caused by an infection or may be idiopathic, as in the case of IBD. Blood with mucus or discharge is found in patients with IBD and carcinoma. In almost all patients with rectal bleeding who are 25–30 years old or older further endoscopic evaluations should be performed. Indications for further investigation in younger patients include significant family history of IBD or cancer, nonresolution of the bleeding after treatment of the condition that is presumed to be the source of bleeding, or bleeding not concomitant with an anorectal source.

Table 7.1 Establishing a diagnosis

Chief complaint	History of present illness
Rectal bleeding	Painful, non-painful, associated with BMs
Anorectal pain	Swelling/non-swelling/associated with BMs
Mass/perianal swelling	IBD, prior abscess
Altered bowel habits	Change in consistency, shape, size and frequency
Constipation	
Diarrhea	
Pruritus Ani	

BMs = bowel movements, IBD = inflammatory bowel disease.
Data from Reference 1.

Table 7.2 Causes of rectal bleeding

Bright red rectal bleeding	Occult blood
Hemorrhoids	Gastritis
Diverticulosis	Gastric ulcer
Ulcerative colitis	Gastric carcinoma
Infectious colitis	Esophageal varices
Polyps	Esophageal tumors
Carcinoma	Duodenal ulcer
Ischemic colitis	Polyps
Fissure	Carcinoma

Data from References 2 and 3.

Pain

Anorectal pain is caused by a wide variety of pathologies; a complete history and physical evaluation will help to narrow the differential diagnosis (Table 7.3). Anal abscesses and fissures commonly cause anorectal pain.[4] Abscesses just under the skin can be identified by swollen, red, tender, areas. Abscesses deeper to the rectum often cause fewer signs but may produce fever and pain in the lower abdomen. Difficulty with bowel evacuation may occur with severe abscesses. Anal fissures are commonly caused by passage of a large, hard stool. This passage is associated with pain, usually described as burning, cutting, or tearing during and after bowel movement.

Table 7.3 Causes of anorectal pain

Anal fissures

Thrombosed external hemorrhoids

Anorectal abscess

Foreign body

Fecal impaction

Neoplasm

Myopathy

Proctalgia fugax

Colonic endometriosis

Prostatitis

Data from Reference 4.

A patient with a thrombosed external hemorrhoid may present with complaints of an acutely painful mass external to the anal opening. The pain usually peaks 48–72 hours after the thrombosis develops, and the symptoms often improve following this as the thrombus dissipates. Sharp rectal pain described by the patient as a spasm is more consistent with proctalgia fugax. Left lower quadrant abdominal pain accompanying hematochezia or diarrhea may be due to IBD, ischemic colitis, or cancer. The use of radiographic imaging and colonoscopy may help elucidate the cause. When obstructive symptoms are present, a neoplasm should be considered. When associated with abdominal distention, a volvulus could also be considered but should be easily recognizable on routine abdominal X-rays.

Masses

Perianal masses are common and represent abscesses, hemorrhoids, anal condyloma, and occasionally a neoplasm. Complete assessment, including a detailed history, inspection, palpation, and anoscopy should be performed. Biopsy, sigmoidoscopy or colonoscopy, may be needed to define the exact nature of the mass.

Pruritus ani

Pruritus ani is a very common symptom and is associated with a wide range of mechanical, dermatologic, infectious, systemic, and other conditions. When pruritus ani becomes chronic, the perianal area becomes lichenified and appears white with fine fissures. Excessive cleaning, and particularly the use of brushes and caustic soaps, aggravates the sensitive tissues and exacerbates the condition. Although older texts emphasized parasitic infestation, this is a rare cause of pruritus ani except for pinworms (*Enterobius vermicularis*) in children.

Fecal impaction

This condition is most commonly seen in those who are inactive or on prolonged bedrest due to surgery, accident, or illness. The elderly in nursing homes and those with chronic constipation are especially at risk. Medications such as narcotics predispose to this problem, and it is a common complication of anorectal procedures as a result of reflex spasm of the anal sphincter. The patient may present with acute abdominal pain or chronic large-bowel obstruction. Paradoxically, patients may have incontinence with diarrhea secondary to a ball valve effect of the fecal bolus. Rectal examination reveals hard, bulky stool in the rectal vault.

Fecal incontinence

Fecal incontinence is the loss of anal sphincter control, leading to the unwanted or untimely release of feces or gas. A thorough history – including duration of fecal incontinence, type of incontinence, frequency of incontinent episodes – and type of stool, impact of the disorder on the patient's life, and history of associated trauma or surgery should be obtained.[5] Specific obstetric history should be obtained, including the use of forceps, tears, and episiotomies associated with vaginal deliveries. Review medications and dietary habits to determine if an easily remedied cause exists. An incontinence score can be used to assess the severity of incontinence and to monitor the results of treatment.[6] A review of systems for systemic medical conditions that contribute to fecal incontinence is important. Asking the patient to keep a diary of the time and frequency of incontinent episodes may be helpful.[6]

Anorectal examination

Anorectal evaluation consists of inspection, palpation, and anoscopic examination, and it can be performed in the prone jackknife or left lateral (Sims) position (Figure 7.2). The knee-chest position is another type of position not usually used. The jackknife position provides the best exposure of the perineum. At Cleveland Clinic Florida (CCF), we examine patients in the prone jackknife position on a Ritter table.

(a)

(b)

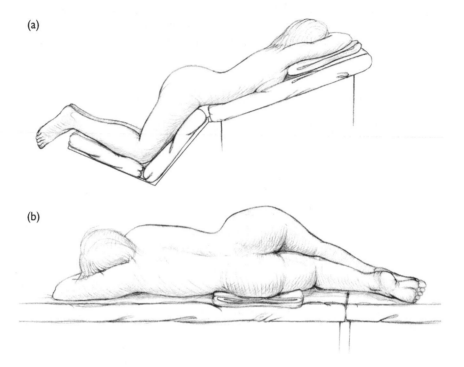

Figure 7.2 Anorectal examination positions: (a) prone (jackknife) position and (b) left lateral (Sims) position.

Inspection

The gluteus muscle or buttocks must be spread to provide adequate visualization of the anus. If necessary, the patient can assist by raising the right gluteal area with the right hand to better expose the perianal area. One should look at the perianal skin and anal verge, which can reveal fissures, fistulae, perianal dermatitis, masses, thrombosed hemorrhoids, condyloma, and other growths. The perianal skin is also examined for any skin changes concomitant with leakage or incontinence. Maneuvers that simulate defecation can identify perineal descent or prolapse. If a full-thickness rectal prolapse is suspected but cannot be reproduced in the prone jackknife position, examination while straining on the toilet bowl can demonstrate the rectal prolapse.

Palpation

Unless the patient is experiencing extreme pain, a digital examination should always be performed. Digital examination is always performed with a lubricated gloved index finger. In males, the prostate should be palpated in addition to digital assessment of the anal canal, and in woman, a bi-digital examination of the rectovaginal (RV) septum is also performed. The finger sweep must include all 360° around the anal canal and distal rectum; any palpable mass must be evaluated further. Because of the redundant mucosa, small rectal tumors may not be visualized with an anoscope but can often be detected by palpation.

The resting pressure should be noted and then the patient should be asked to squeeze. This will provide further information about the integrity of the external sphincter and puborectalis muscle.

Anoscopy

Anoscopy is the final step in the initial office examination, and it permits evaluation of the anal canal. Many types of anoscopes are available, but the most commonly used at CCF is the Barr–Shuford (Figure 7.3). A lubricant is applied to the entire instrument, and it should be inserted gently. The introducer is removed and one-quarter of the mucosa is visualized as the anoscope is slowly removed. The instrument is then rotated 90° and rein-serted. This is done four times to visualize the entire circumference of the anal canal. Anoscopes may also allow visualization of distal rectal mucosa.

Flexible sigmoidoscopy

Flexible sigmoidoscopy is an important diagnostic screening procedure because its ability to visualize the rectum and distal colon. The 60-cm flexible sigmoidoscope provides excellent visualization with minimal discomfort to patients, compared to the rigid sigmoidoscopy, which is uncomfortable, shorter, and less rewarding. Sigmoidoscopy can identify 55% of colorectal cancers as they are within the length of the sigmoido-scope.[7] Flexible sigmoidoscopy is indicated for screening for colorectal carcinomas or polyps, but mostly to evaluate anorectal complaints in the office.[8] Complete colonic evaluation is accomplished via colonoscopy.

Approach

Preparations before flexible sigmoidoscopy consist of 2 Fleet™ enemas before examination.[9] The patient is placed on the examination table in the left lateral position with knees drawn to the chest or in the prone jack-knife position. After the digital examination, the lubricated flexible

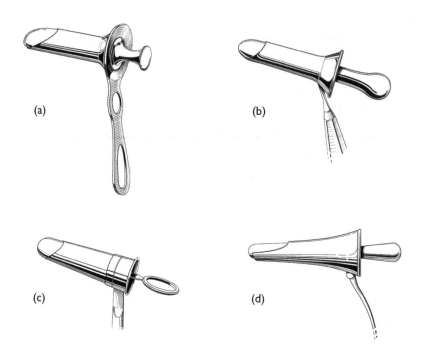

Figure 7.3 Different types and sizes of anoscopes with obturators are useful for evaluation of the anal canal and may be inserted before examination with the flexible sigmoidoscope: (a) Hirschman 2.5 inch (5.7 cm); (b) Mod Martin 22 × 75 mm; (c) Bensuade 22 mm; and (d) Barr–Shuford 4.5 inch (11.4 cm). The most frequently used anoscope at the Cleveland Clinic Florida is the Barr–Shuford 4.5 inch (11.4 cm).

sigmoidoscope is introduced into the rectum, where it is advanced under direct vision, keeping the lumen in view at all times. The scope should not be advanced against resistance. Overdistention of the bowel with air should be avoided, because it produces discomfort to the patient and makes intubation more difficult. The colon is best inspected as the scope is withdrawn after full advancement. At this time, the lumen and folds of the colon should be examined for pathology. Once the scope has been withdrawn to the level of the rectum, it should be retroflexed to look down; also known as the *J* maneuver, this provides an opportunity to view the distal area of the rectum, which is difficult to observe during insertion.[10] Flexible sigmoidoscopy is a safe procedure, with a very low percentage of complications.[11] Perforation of the colon is rare; in a series by Marks and associates, one perforation occurred in 1012 examinations.[12]

Radiologic evaluation

Computed tomography

Computed tomography (CT) has also proven disappointing. The exact site of pathology in relation to the levators on axial CT scans can only be inferred indirectly through the relation of any abnormality to the piriformis and coccygeus muscles. The levators are not well identified, and sphincter resolution is poor. Coronal imaging is rarely possible and there are many pitfalls in interpretation of the images. The value of CT in the initial work-up of anorectal disorders is limited.[13] However, CT is helpful in defining the extent of rectocecal tumors or cysts and may offer information regarding processes in the perirectal fat, adjacent organs, and the pelvis.

Magnetic resonance imaging

Patients with deep anorectal abscess may be better studied with magnetic resonance imaging (MRI). Accuracy of MRI is higher than digital examination in determining the presence of ischiorectal or pelvirectal abscess, particularly when they occur at the same time. The sensitivity and specificity for detecting fistula tracts were 100% and 86%, respectively; abscesses, 96% and 97%, respectively; horseshoe fistulas, 100% and 100%, respectively; and internal openings, 96% and 90%, respectively. Magnetic resonance imaging is accurate for detecting anal fistulas and provides important additional information in patients with Crohn's disease-related and recurrent anal fistulas.[14] MRI and hydrogen peroxide-enhanced three-dimensional endoanal ultrasound have good agreement for classification of the primary fistula tract and the location of an internal opening and they are both reliable methods for preoperative evaluation.[15] Compared with endoanal ultrasound, endoanal MRI more accurately allows depiction and classification of fistulas.[16]

Endoanal ultrasound

Endoanal ultrasound can be applied in the management of fecal incontinence, rectal tumors, and inflammatory perianal conditions. In fecal incontinence, anal ultrasound will confirm the presence or absence of sphincter defects and is also important to diagnose complex anorectal abscesses and fistula (Figure 7.4). In the detection and staging of rectal cancer, transrectal ultrasound (TRUS) is an important tool, since it enables the distinction of various layers of rectal wall.[17] Men may be examined in the left lateral position, but women always should be examined in the prone position, because better views of the perineum are obtained.[18] With the TRUS, rectal tumors can be staged according to the TNM classification (Table 7.4). The accuracy of TRUS ranges between 67% and 93%.[19,20]

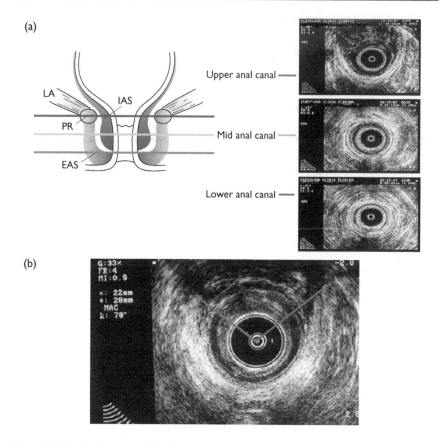

Figure 7.4 Anal ultrasound showing (a) normal architecture of the anal canal and (b) EAS, IAS defect in the anterior quadrant.
EAS = external anal sphincter, IAS = internal anal sphincter, PR = puborectalis.

Table 7.4 Transrectal ultrasound staging system

Level	Description
T1	Tumors confined to the mucosa and submucosa
T2	Tumors invading the proper muscle layer, but confined to rectal wall
T3	Tumors penetrating the perirectal fat
T4	Invasion into adjacent organs
N0	No lymph node metastases
N1	Lymph node metastases

Physiologic examinations

Anal continence and bowel evacuation is a complicated evaluation in which there is no single test that can provide a full detailed description. Anal manometry, defecography, and electromyography (EMG) are used in conjunction to evaluate anorectal functions, especially in patients suffering from fecal incontinence, constipation, and pelvic floor disorders.

Anal manometry

The purpose of anal manometry is to evaluate the integrated function of the defecation unit, including its motor and sensory function. Anorectal manometry can define functional weakness of one or both sphincter muscles by providing information on resting pressure, squeezing pressure, high-pressure zone (HPZ), and rectoanal inhibitory relfex (RAIR). Multichannel catheters can be used to assess the entire length of the anal canal in all directions. Anal manometry is recognized to be the least accurate and helpful of the physiologic tests. It is complimentary in the assessment of sphincter injury and failed overlapping sphincteroplasty.[21,22]

Electromyography and pudendal nerve terminal motor latency

Anorectal EMGs consist of measurements of pudendal nerve terminal motor latency (PNTML), assessing the conduction time in the pudendal nerve from Alcock's canal to the end organ in the external sphincter. Findings reflect the myelin function of the peripheral nerve, and the test allows for the evaluation of pelvic floor neuromuscular integrity. The pudendal nerve is stimulated at the ischial spine transanally. The latency period between stimulation of the nerve and evoked response of the muscle is measured. Any damage to the neuromuscular unit results in the prolongation of the latency. Normal latency has been described as 2 ms ($\pm$ 0.2 ms). Prolonged times suggest injury to the large fast-conducting fibers.[23] Abnormal findings after EMG evaluation are present in more than 90% of patients with fecal incontinence. Ryhammer and colleagues evaluated the long-term effects of vaginal delivery on anorectal function and found that PNTML increased with parity.[24] Prolonged latencies may be associated with obstetric injury, prolapse, perineal descent, and neuropathies. Pudendal neuropathy is observed in 70% of patient with fecal incontinence, and over 50% of patients with sphincter injury.[25]

Cinedefecography

Cinedefecography provides pelvic dynamic measurements during evacuation, and consequently provides enough information for the diagnosis of functional disorders such as paradoxical puborectalis contraction and excessive perineal descent, and also assesses anatomic abnormalities such as rectocele, enterocele, and rectoanal intussusception. Cinedefecography is a very helpful tool that can also evaluate rectal emptying, which may help to differentiate an anatomic finding from a physiologic disorder.[26]

References

1. Perry WB. History and physical examination. In: Beck DE, ed. Handbook of Colorectal Surgery. St Louis: Quality Medical Publishing 1997:30–8
2. Nelson RL, Abcarian H, Davis FG, et al. Prevalence of benign anorectal disease in a randomly selected population. Dis Colon Rectum 1995;38(4):341–4.
3. Helfand M, Marton KI, Zimmer-Gembeck MJ, Sox HC. History of visible rectal bleeding in primary care population. Initial assessment and 10-year follow-up. JAMA 1997;277:44–8.
4. Ger GC, Wexner SD, Jorge JM, et al. Evaluation and treatment of chronic intractable rectal pain. Dis Colon Rectum 1993;36(2):139–45.
5. Jorge JM, Wexner SD. Etiology and management of fecal incontinence. Dis Colon Rectum 1993;36(1):77–97.
6. Rockwood TH, Church JM, Fleshman JW, et al. Fecal Incontinence Quality of life instrument for patients with fecal incontinence. Dis Colon Rectum 2000; 43(1):9–16.
7. Winawer SJ, Leidner SD, Boyle C, et al. Comparison of flexible sigmoidoscopy with other diagnostic techniques in the diagnosis of rectocolon neoplasia. Dig Dis Sci 1979;24:277–81.
8. Montano DE, Selby JV, Somkin CP, Bhat A, Nadel M. Acceptance of flexible sigmoidoscopy screening for colorectal cancer. Cancer Detect Prev 2004;28(1): 43–51.
9. Crespi M, Casale V, Grassi A. Flexible sigmoidoscopy. Surg Clin North Am 1980;60:465–79.
10. Blom J, Liden A, Nilsson J, et al. Colorectal cancer screening with flexible sigmoidoscopy – participant's experience and technical feasibility. Eur J Surg Oncol 2004;30(4):362–9.
11. Opelka FG. Transanal endoscopy. In: Hicks TC, Beck DE, Opelka FG, Timmcke AE, eds. Complications of Colon and Rectal Surgery. Baltimore: Williams & Wilkins, 1996:143–52.
12. Marks G, Boggs HW, Catro AF, et al. Sigmoidoscopic examinations with rigid and flexible fiberoptic sigmoidoscopes in the surgeon's office: a comparative prospective study of effectiveness in 1012. Dis Colon Rectum 1979;22:162–8.
13. Horton KM, Abrahms RA, Fishman EK. Spiral CT of colon cancer: imaging features and role of management. Radiographics 2000;20:419–30.
14. Beets-Tan RG, Beets GL, van der Hoop AG, et al. Preoperative MR imaging of anal fistulas: Does it really help the surgeon? Radiology 2001;218(1):75–84.

15. West RL, Zimmerman DD, Dwarskasing S, et al. Prospective comparison of hydrogen peroxide-enhanced three-dimensional endoanal ultrasonography and endoanal magnetic resonance imaging of perianal fistulas. Dis Colon Rectum 2003;46(10):1407–15.

16. Hussain SM, Stoker J, Schouten WR, et al. Fistula in ano: endoanal sonography versus endoanal MR imaging in classification. Radiology 1996;200(2):475–81.

17. Heriot AG, Grundy A, Kumar D. Preoperative staging of rectal carcinoma. Br J Surg 1999;86:17–28.

18. Frudinger A, Bartram CI, Halligan S, et al. Examination techniques for endosonography of the anal canal. Abdom Imaging 1998;23:301–3.

19. Solomon MJ, McLeod RS. Endoluminal trans rectal ultrasonography: accuracy, reliability, and validity. Dis Colon Rectum 1993;36(2):200–5.

20. Beynon J. An evaluation of the role of rectal endosonography in rectal cancer. Ann R Coll Surg Engl 1989;71:131–9.

21. Sentovich SM, Blatchford GJ, Rivela LJ, et al. Diagnosing anal sphincter injury with TAUS and manometry. Dis Colon Rectum 1997;40:1430–4.

22. Ternent CA, Shashidharan M, Blatchford GJ, et al. Transanal ultrasound and anorectal physiology findings affecting continence after sphincteroplasty. Dis Colon Rectum 1997;40:462–7.

23. Kiff ES, Swash M. Slowed conduction in the pudendal nerves in idiopathic (neurogenic) fecal incontinence. Br J Surg 1984;71:614–16.

24. Ryhammer AM, Laurberg S, Hermann AP. Long-term effect of vaginal deliveries on anorectal function in normal perimenopausal women. Dis Colon Rectum 1996;39(8):852–9.

25. Roig JV, Villoslada C, Lledo S, et al. Prevalence of pudendal neuropathy in fecal incontinence. Results of a prospective study. Dis Colon Rectum 1995;38(9):952–8.

26. Johansson C, Nilsson BY, Holmstrom B, et al. Association between rectocele and paradoxical sphincter response. Dis Colon Rectum 1992;35:503–9.

Chapter 8

Urodynamics

Gamal Ghoniem and Usama Khater

Introduction

Urodynamic investigation is a functional assessment of the lower urinary tract to provide an objective pathophysiologic explanation for the symptoms and dysfunction of the urinary tract. Urodynamic studies comprise a series of tests, and the appropriate test should be selected and performed in an attempt to answer a question on the target function to be evaluated. The information provided by urodynamic studies may be useful in establishing the etiology of the dysfunction and may help in selecting the most appropriate intervention. Prior to urodynamic investigation, a medical history, physical examination, and voiding diary should be obtained, as such information is necessary in order to select the appropriate studies and anticipate which events might take place during the urodynamic investigation. Unfortunately, urodynamic testing is not a set of laboratory values like blood chemistry values, but rather a physiologic testing that may be affected by several factors. Presence of the clinician during the studies is essential for successful interpretation of findings.

Uroflowmetry

Uroflowmetry is the measurement of the rate of urine flow over time. It is the most commonly used form of urodynamic studies and performed as an initial screening test when voiding dysfunction is suspected. The results may then prompt further investigations. Uroflowmetry is performed by having the patient void on a special commode that funnels the urine onto a device that measures the volume voided over time. There are various measurement techniques used by the uroflowmeters such as the rotating disk method, electronic dip, weight transducers, and graphimetric method. The rotating disk method is the most common method; the voided volume is directed onto a rotating disk and the amount landing on the disk produces a proportionate increase in its inertia. The power required to keep the disk rotating at a constant rate is measured, thus allowing the calculation of the flow rate. Privacy, voided volume, patient age, and sex are factors affecting the parameters of uroflowmetry. The uroflowmetric parameters to be recorded and reported include total voided volume (V), maximum flow rate (Q_{max}), time to Q_{max}, voiding time (V_t), flow time, and average flow rate (Q_{ave}). The pattern of the flow curve is also observed.[1] In young males, Q_{max} should be 15–25 ml/s. Women typically void with a slightly higher maximum flow (5–10 ml/s) for a given volume than men.[2] A normal flow pattern or curve is a continuous bell-shaped smooth curve (Figure 8.1). The first 45% of voided volume is reached before Q_{max} is reached. The overall appearance of the flow curve may disclose abnormalities. This is commonly due to abnormal straining superimposed on detrusor contraction. An interrupted pattern is consistent with intermittent flow in which downward deflection reaches 2 ml/s or lower. The obstructed flow is characterized by prolonged flow time, sustained low flow rate, low Q_{max}, low Q_{ave}, and a plateau-shaped curve (Figure 8.2). There is slow initial rise with an increased time to

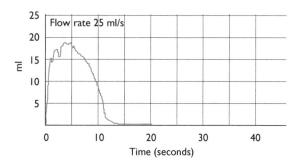

Figure 8.1 Normal flow pattern.

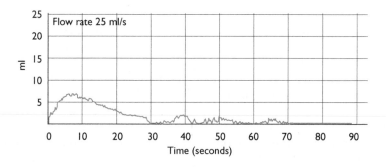

Figure 8.2 Obstructed flow in 70-year-old male patient with obstructing benign prostatic hyperplasia.

achieve Q_{max}, but because the voiding time is longer, Q_{max} may be seen relatively earlier.[3]

The flow pattern of a patient with urethral obstruction is a flat-topped curve with decreased Q_{max}, which is quickly reached but remains at the same level for most of micturition. The curve is unbroken and flattened with a large part of the volume voided at a constant Q_{max}[4] (Figure 8.3).

The urinary flow rate provides useful information about whether there is obstruction to the outflow tract, especially in males. A flow rate greater than 40 ml/s is considered superflow, which is common in women and may be due to decreased outlet resistance.[5] It is particularly seen in women who have genuine stress urinary incontinence (SUI), where the outlet resistance is much reduced, and in patients with marked bladder activity. Although low Q_{max} may indicate urinary outlet obstruction, measurement of the flow rate alone has limited value, as it can be seen in impaired detrusor contractility.

Post-void residual volume (PVR) is the volume in the bladder immediately after voiding is completed. It is an excellent assessment of bladder emptying, and it reflects bladder contractility. When it is combined with PVR, uroflowmetry can be a good screening tool for voiding dysfunction. PVR can be measured by ultrasound or catheterization immediately after voiding and, in an adult, it can be up to 25 ml; a residual volume more than 100 ml warrants surveillance.[6] Residual volume may be overestimated in patients with vesicoureteral reflux, hydroureteronephrosis, and bladder diverticulum. When a normal Q_{max} and normal voided volume without residual urine are present, infravesical obstruction or reduced contractility is unlikely. Several nomograms have been used to interpret the measured flow rates. Siroky's nomogram is used for males, and the Liverpool nomograms have scales for males and females. A peak flow over the 90th percentile on the Liverpool nomogram may be suspicious for detrusor overactivity.[7]

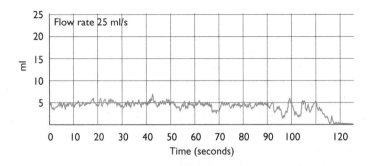

Figure 8.3 Obstructed flow pattern in 50-year-old patient with urethral stricture.

Cystometry

Cystometry is a measure of the bladder pressure response to filling. A cystometrogram (CMG) is a graphic presentation of pressure as a function of volume; the x-axis represents volume and the y-axis represents pressure. Filling CMG is an excellent representation of the passive properties of the detrusor (i.e. viscoelastic properties). Several parameters are provided by this study: bladder filling sensation, stability, compliance, capacity, control over micturition, detrusor contractility, and emptying.

Single-channel cystometry

Cystometry can be performed as a single-channel study in which the pressure within the bladder, which is the intravesical pressure (P_{ves}), is measured during filling and storage. It consists of a Foley catheter in the bladder attached to a wide-mouthed syringe without plunger and held at the level of the superior edge of the pubic symphysis. Saline is incrementally poured in the syringe and thus retrograde into the bladder. The height of the column of saline indicates the pressure of the tonic segment of the cystometric curve. A detrusor contraction during any part of bladder filling results in a rapid rise in the column of saline or water. With this technique the monitored pressure is the intravesical pressure (P_{ves}). This reflects the cumulative effects of all sources of pressure on the bladder – namely, intra-abdominal pressure, which is the pressure surrounding the bladder, and detrusor pressure (the pressure derived from bladder wall smooth muscle activity, active and passive). With a single-channel recording system, it is difficult to ascertain the exact source of the rise in intravesical pressure, either due to detrusor contraction or increased intra-abdominal pressure (cough or patient movement). To distinguish the source of the rise of P_{ves}, multichannel cystometry should be performed.

Multichannel cystometry

In a multichannel study, concurrent measurement of intravesical, abdominal, and urethral pressures is performed (Figure 8.4). Detrusor pressure is estimated by subtracting abdominal pressure from intravesical pressure. The electromyography (EMG) is also monitored.

Intravesical pressure (P_{ves}) represents the total pressures acting upon the bladder, detrusor (P_{det}), and abdominal pressures (P_{abd}) (Figure 8.5). Detrusor pressure is a component of intravesical pressure that is created by forces in the bladder wall, passive and active. The passive forces are produced by the viscoelastic property of the bladder wall, and active forces are created by detrusor contraction and tone. Exterior forces act upon the bladder by the abdominal pressure.

$$P_{ves} = P_{det} + P_{abd}$$

then

$$P_{det} = P_{ves} - P_{abd}$$

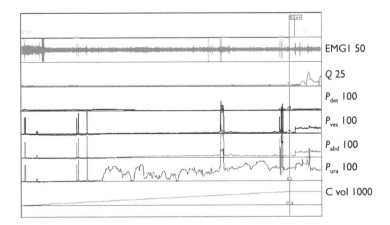

Figure 8.4 Multichannel cystometry showing a normal cystometrogram. (See also color image on p. xxiv)

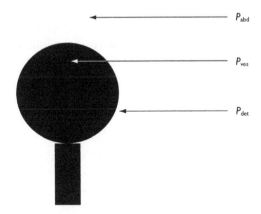

Figure 8.5 Urodynamic algebra. P_{abd} = abdominal pressure, P_{ves} = intravesical pressure, P_{det} = detrusor pressure.

Therefore in a nearly empty bladder, $P_{det} = 0$, so in this situation, $P_{ves} = P_{abd}$ (P_{abd} may be slightly greater than P_{ves} because of the rectal balloon compliance).

For cystometry studies, urodynamic laboratories use different instruments and techniques. There are different catheters, such as microtip, air-charged, fiberoptic, and water-infused. Intravesical pressure (P_{ves}) is measured by placing a catheter into the bladder to fill and detect the pressure. The catheter may have two lumens: one for filling and the other for pressure monitoring. A triple-lumen catheter is used when urethral pressure is simultaneously monitored. Abdominal pressure is measured by using a rectal balloon catheter, as the rectum and bladder are in close proximity and the intra-abdominal pressure experienced by both organs is equal. Vaginal pressure monitoring can be used in women, but the vagina is subject to many anatomic changes that may alter pressure transmission; however, it can be used if there are anatomic changes of the rectum. Historically, both liquid and gas have been used as a filling medium. Gas is a rapid and inexpensive filling medium. However, it is unphysiologic, compressible, and easily provokes detrusor overactivity. It is not suitable for studying voiding and leakage. Gas is seldom now used as a filling medium. The liquid filling medium may be saline, water, or radiographic contrast. The bladder can be filled either antegrade or retrograde: the latter is used more commonly in the office setting because of time consideration. The temperature of the liquid is either room temperature or body temperature. According to the International Continence Society (ICS), the filling rate is considered fast (>100 ml/min), medium (10–100 ml/min), or slow (<10 ml/min).[6] Natural bladder filling is on average 1–2 ml/min. Rapid infusion may induce involuntary contractions or give the appearance of decreased compliance. A rapid infusion rate is used to provoke occult detrusor overactivity.[8] Slow infusion is used for children and adults with small functional capacity or unusual sensitivity to filling at medium filling rate.

Interpretation of cystometry

Bladder capacity

There are different bladder capacities. Functional capacity is the average volume of urine voided during the day. The ICS recommends the voiding diary for its measurement. Anatomic capacity, which is obtained during endoscopic examination with the patient sedated or under anesthesia, is the volume at which a patient who has normal sensation feels that he/she can no longer delay micturition. In absence of sensation, it is the volume at which the clinician decides to terminate filling. The cystometric capacity in an adult should be 300–600 ml. Women have a greater bladder capacity than men.

An enlarged bladder capacity is seen in patients with chronic distention and sensory or motor impairment. Smaller capacity may be found in patients who have sensory urgency, unstable detrusor contractions, infection or inflammation, or following bladder surgery or radiation. It is related to low compliance.

Compliance

Compliance is the change in volume with pressure and is expressed in ml/cmH$_2$O. It represents the bladder distensibility and is attributed to the viscoelastic property and the spherical shape of the bladder. Also, the absence of involuntary contractions during filling contributes to the bladder compliance. As a result, the detrusor pressure remains low throughout bladder filling. Normally, while the bladder is filling, the detrusor pressure does not exceed 5–10 cmH$_2$O above the starting pressure. Therefore, the kidneys are protected and continence is assured. The cystometrogram is divided into four phases.

The compliance is calculated at the end of filling:

$$\text{Compliance} = \Delta \text{ Volume} / \Delta P_{det}$$

According to Ghoniem, the compliance in the normal individual is ≥20 ml/cmH$_2$O.[9] Compliance less than 10 ml/cmH$_2$O is clinically significant. Low compliance is found in patients with severe outlet obstruction, meningomyelocele, chronic inflammation such as tuberculosis and following radiotherapy. High compliance may be associated with a large capacity and overdistended bladders. It has little clinical significance as an isolated finding.

Sensation of the bladder

The sensation part of cystometry is subjective and variable. The sensitivity and functional capacity are best determined through voiding diaries and not by cystometry. The first sensation is the first awareness of filling and is considerably variable. Many patients describe a filling sensation immediately. Typically, the first sensation to urinate is felt at 90–150 ml. The normal desire to void is the feeling that leads the patient to pass urine at the next convenient moment, but voiding can be delayed if necessary. Strong desire to void is felt when there is a persistent urge to void without the fear of leakage. Urgency is a strong desire to void accompanied by fear of leakage or pain. Urgency is usually felt at 200–400 ml and bladder fullness usually occurs at 300–600 ml. Pain during bladder filling or micturition is abnormal.

Early sensation of filling (sensory urgency) may indicate inflammation, unstable detrusor contractions, or decreased bladder compliance. Delayed sensation of filling may represent a neurologic disorder such as peripheral neuropathy of the pelvic plexus, trauma, or disease affecting the sacral nerves.

Stability

Normally, the bladder stores increasing volumes of urine without a significant rise in pressure due to the compliance and absence of involuntary detrusor contractions. The only time that the bladder should contract is during the voluntary act of voiding. Under certain circumstances, the bladder may show involuntary contractions, which may be associated with symptoms. These involuntary contractions are divided into two categories by the ICS: idiopathic and neurogenic detrusor overactivities. Idiopathic detrusor overactivity is defined as involuntary contractions not associated with an underlying neurologic lesion. The cause of this overactivity may be idiopathic, aging, infection, inflammation, or bladder outlet obstruction. Neurogenic detrusor overactivity is defined as the involuntary contractions associated with a known neurologic lesion and is seen in upper motor neuron lesions. Idiopathic and neurogenic detrusor overactivity may look identical on the CMG. The terms idiopathic and neurogenic overactivity are strictly defined by the patient's neurologic status rather than the appearance on the CMG. Absence of involuntary contractions does not exclude its existence, especially if the patient's symptoms are not reproduced during the testing. Involuntary detrusor contractions have been recorded in normal subjects without any voiding symptoms.

Rectal contractions

Rectal contractions may occur during multichannel urodynamic studies. They were previously considered artifacts or variants of normal. Combs and Nitti reported that rectal contractions occur more frequently in patients with voiding dysfunction.[10] Ghoniem et al found rectal contractions in 40% of patients with symptomatic benign prostatic hyperplasia (BPH) and detrusor overactivity and in 10% of symptomatic BPH patients without detrusor overactivity; the difference was statistically significant.[11]

Stress-induced detrusor instability

Increased abdominal pressure by cough may trigger uninhibited detrusor contractions in some patients. If they are associated with incontinence, the leakage occurs due to these contractions and not due to the increased abdominal pressure itself. This phenomenon is responsible for 7% of women with stress incontinence.[10]

Pressure–flow studies

Pressure–flow studies are simultaneous measurements of detrusor pressure and urine flow rate. They provide more accurate and useful information than uroflow rate alone. The major reason for these studies is to diagnose outlet obstruction and distinguish obstruction versus impaired detrusor contraction. Approximately 20–35 cmH$_2$O of pressure is required to drive urine across the normal male urethra.[12] Women void with lower detrusor contraction and pressure and higher flows than men.[13] Detrusor pressures greater than 30 cmH$_2$O tend to indicate the presence of some degree of obstruction. There are no generally accepted pressure–flow criteria for obstruction in women. Massey and Abrams defined bladder outlet obstruction at Q_{max} <12 ml/s and $P_{det}Q_{max}$ >50 cmH$_2$O, urethral resistance ($P_{det}Q_{max}/Q_{max}$) >0.2, and 'significant' residual urine.[14] Farrar et al used an arbitrary definition based on Q_{max} <15 m/s and $P_{det}Q_{max}$ >50 cmH$_2$O.[15] Chassagne et al reported that Q_{max} ≤ 15 ml/s and $P_{det}Q_{max}$ >20 cmH$_2$O are reasonable pressure–flow parameters to define female bladder outlet obstruction (BOO).[16] Blaivas and Groutz constructed a nomogram for women with obstructive urinary symptoms.[17]

The results of pressure–flow studies can be classified according to a number of nomograms. Most of these nomograms have been described in men because of the prevalence of bladder outlet obstruction. The drawback of these nomograms is the presence of a broad boundary between obstruction and non-obstruction.[18]

Leak point pressure

Historically, the leak point pressure was introduced by McGuire as a method to predict which children with myelodysplasia were at increased risk of upper urinary tract impairment because of the chronically elevated pressure. The leak point pressure is the bladder pressure at which leakage occurs. The rise in bladder pressure causing this leakage may originate either from the detrusor or from increase in abdominal pressure. Therefore, two leak point pressures have been described – the bladder or detrusor leak point pressure (DLPP) and the abdominal leak point pressure (ALPP). Each measures the closure function of the entire bladder outlet under different circumstances. ALPP is the intravesical pressure at which urine leakage occurs due to increased abdominal pressure in the absence of detrusor contraction. The increase in abdominal pressure can be produced during the study by asking the patient to cough (CLPP) or to do Valsalva maneuver (VLPP). Although coughing can produce higher abdominal pressures, Valsalva maneuver produces better-controlled abdominal pressure. If Valsalva maneuver failed to detect leakage, CLPP can be done.

The DLPP is the value of detrusor pressure at which leaks occur in the absence of an abdominal pressure rise. DLPP was introduced in myelodysplastic children as an indicator of the risk of upper tract deterioration. McGuire and Ghoniem reported that DLPP exceeding 40 cmH$_2$O with low compliance is associated with imminent risk of upper urinary tract damage.[19] ALPP less than 90 cmH$_2$O suggests intrinsic sphincter deficiency (ISD).[20–22]

Urethral pressure profile

Urethral pressure profile (UPP) is a measure of urethral resistance along the urethral lumen. The measurement can be made at one point in the urethra over a period of time or several points along the length of urethra. There are three techniques used for measuring the UPP:

- perfusion method
- catheter-mounted transducers
- air-charged balloon catheter profilometry.

The perfusion method is the most widely used. Intravesical pressure should be measured to exclude a simultaneous detrusor contraction and to calculate the closing pressure. The intraluminal pressure can be determined at rest, with the bladder at any given volume, during cough or during voiding. The principle of measuring stress UPP (during cough) is to measure pressure transmission from the abdominal cavity to the urethra. In stress incontinence, this pressure transmission is inadequate and the urethral closure pressure becomes negative with coughing. Voiding urethral pressure is used to determine the pressure and site of urethral obstruction. This technique is plagued by artifacts secondary to movement of the catheter. Relevant measurements relating to resting UPP include maximal urethral pressure (MUP), maximal urethral closure pressure (MUCP), and functional urethral length. The maximum pressure measured is the MUP. The maximum difference between urethral pressure and the intravesical pressure is MUCP. The functional profile length is the length of the urethra along which the urethral pressure exceeds intravesical pressure in women. The pressure transmission ratio is the increment in urethral pressure on stress as a percentage of the simultaneously recorded increment in intravesical pressure.

The drawback of UPP is that there are no defined normal values for UPP, as considerable variations have been reported. Although MUCP tends to be lower in women with genuine stress incontinence, there is overlap between SUI patients and normal subjects. Other drawbacks of UPP are its difficulty to standardize and perform and its lack of correlation with the surgical outcome. Also, the correlation between the severity of stress incontinence and low MUCP has limited relevance.[23] While UPP has limited applications because of inter- and intra-individual variations, it is used to diagnose the ISD or 'low-pressure urethra'.

Intrinsic sphincter deficiency

Poor function of the internal sphincter is referred to as intrinsic sphincter deficiency (ISD). McGuire recognized this condition in some women with recurrent SUI and with low urethral closing pressure. He defined that condition as SUI type III. Pure ISD is easy to diagnose, as the urethra is fixed and incontinence occurs with low pressure. It is often seen after multiple failed incontinence surgeries or radiation therapy. The ALPP is used to determine if ISD exists in the presence of urethral hypermobility. It is generally accepted that proximal urethral closing pressure less than 10 cmH$_2$O and ALPP of 60 cmH$_2$O or less indicate ISD. There is a gray zone between 60 and 90 cmH$_2$O. Ghoniem classified ISD into three subgroups based on videofluorourodynamic (VFUD) findings and ALPP (Table 8.1). ISD-A is diagnosed only by VFUD, as the bladder neck is not open at rest and it is difficult to diagnose radiographically (Figure 8.6). ISD-B is characterized by a peak-shaped open bladder neck at rest (Figure 8.7). The ALPP is less than 90 cmH$_2$O. ISD-C is characterized by an open, fixed nonfunctioning urethra (pipestem) with high position of the bladder neck (Figure 8.8); the ALPP is less than 70 cmH$_2$O.[24]

Videourodynamics

Videourodynamics is a combination of a routine urodynamic study with X-ray or ultrasound imaging. Videourodynamics/ fluorourodynamics (FUDS) is used for patients with complicated lower urinary tract dysfunction. In patients with neurologic conditions and lower urinary tract dysfunction, videourodynamics may offer a more accurate diagnosis. Because of the invasiveness, radiation exposure, and high initial and running costs, FUDS should not be considered as a first-line evaluation.

Table 8.1 Classification of intrinsic sphincter deficiency (ISD)

Parameter	ISD-A	ISD-B	ISD-C
Stress test	± ve	Mostly +ve	Always +ve
Bladder neck at FUDS	Closed at rest, open with stress	Peak-shaped, open at rest	Pipestem, open at rest
ALPP (cmH$_2$O)	<120	<90	<70

FUDS = fluorourodynamics, ALPP = abdominal leak point pressure.

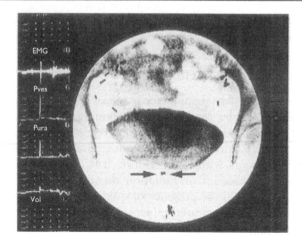

Figure 8.6 ISD-A.

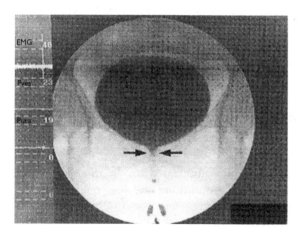

Figure 8.7 ISD-B.

Indications for videourodynamics include neurogenic lower urinary tract dysfunction and incontinence. In these patients, FUDS may define the cause of incontinence when simple urodynamic studies do not lead to a definite diagnosis or after failure of initial therapy based on less-complicated methods of diagnosis.

The advantages of videourodynamics stem from the simultaneous measurement of the pressure and visualization of the anatomy. Videourodynamics may reveal the following:

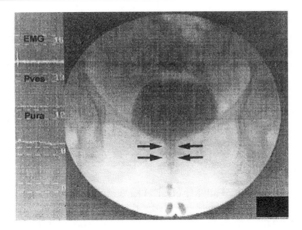

Figure 8.8 ISD-C.

- incompetent bladder neck
- inadequate urethral closure during filling
- location of urethral obstruction during voiding
- descent of the bladder base
- bladder base hypermobility
- intrinsic sphincter deficiency
- incontinence as a leakage of contrast medium, which is demonstrated fluoroscopically
- dyssynergia between detrusor and external sphincter or bladder neck can be documented
- any sign of reflux during the filling or voiding phase can be detected immediately
- bladder or urethral diverticulum or other anatomic malformations.

Electromyography

Electromyography (EMG) is the study of electrical activities generated by the muscle. It provides useful information on sphincter function, but is most valuable when performed with cystometry. To detect these activities, either surface electrodes or needle electrodes are used. Although direct needle electromyography of the urethral sphincter provides the most accurate information, surface electrodes are generally used. EMG recordings show the activity of the voluntary component of the urinary sphincter mechanism and the overall activity of the pelvic floor. The interpretation is mainly restricted to recording of progressively increasing EMG activity during filling of the bladder (guarding reflex). If the EMG activity is reduced or silent during bladder filling, this may indicate an incompetent urethral closure mechanism. Normally, the EMG activity should decrease during voluntary voiding; if this is not the case, urethral function may be overactive. Increased EMG activity during voiding may indicate abdominal straining. Waxing and waning of the sphincter EMG during voiding suggests a functional obstruction (detrusor-sphincter dyssynergia). Surface EMG techniques are also valuable in judging the effect of pelvic floor training therapy and can be used in biofeedback treatment.

References

1. Abrams P, Cardozo L, Fall M, et al. The standardisation of terminology in lower urinary tract function: report from the Standardisation Sub-committee of the International Continence Society. Neurourol Urodyn 2002;21:167–78.
2. Drach G, Ignatoff J, Layton T. Peak urinary flow rate: observations in female subjects and comparison to male subjects. J Urol 1979;122:215–19.
3. Abrams P, Torrens M. Urine flow studies. Urol Clin North Am 1979;6:71–9.
4. Jorgensen J, Jensen K. Uroflowmetry. Urol Clin North Am 1996;23:237–42.
5. Andersen J, Jacobsen O, Gammeigard P, et al. Dysfunction of the bladder neck: a urodynamic study. Urol Int 1976;31:78.
6. Homma Y, Batista J, Bauer S, et al. Urodynamics. In: Incontinence, 2nd International Consultation on Incontinence, July 1–3, 2001, 2nd edn. Plymouth, UK: Health Publications Ltd, 2002;342.
7. Webb R, Griffith C, Ramsden P, et al. Measurement of voiding pressures on ambulatory monitoring: comparison with conventional cystometry. Br J Urol 1990;65:152–4.
8. Susset JG, Ghoniem GM, Regnier CH. Clinical value of rapid cystometrogram in males. Neurourol Urodyn 1982;1:319–27.
9. Ghoniem G. Disorders of bladder compliance. In: Krus E, McGuire E, eds. Female Urology. Philadelphia: Lippincott, 1994.
10. Combs AJ, Nitti V. Significance of rectal contractions noted on multichannel urodynamics. Neurol Urodyn 1995;14:73–80.
11. Ghoniem GM, Khater U, El Segany R, Sakr M. The significance of rectal contractions in benign prostatic obstruction. Urodinamica, 2005;15(1):33–8.
12. McGuire E. Urodynamic studies in prostatic obstruction. In: Fitzpatrick J, Krane R, eds. The Prostate. New York: Churchill Livingstone, 1989:103–9.
13. Ghoniem G. Urodynamics. In: Levy A, ed. Urology pearls of wisdom. Boston: Boston Medical Publishing, 2001:113–18.
14. Massey JA, Abrams PH. Obstructed voiding in the female. Br J Urol 1988;16(1):36–9.
15. Farrar DJ, Osborne JL, Stephen TP, et al. A urodynamic view of bladder outflow obstruction in the female: factors influencing the results of treatment. Br J Urol 1976;47:815–22.
16. Chassagne S, Bernier PA, Haab F, et al. Proposed cutoff values to define bladder outlet obstruction in women. Urology 1998;51:408–11.
17. Blaivas JG, Groutz A. Bladder outlet obstruction nomogram for women with lower urinary tract symptomatology. Neurourol Urodyn 2000;19:553–64.

18. Abrams P, Griffith D. The assessment of prostatic obstruction from uro-dynamic measurements and from residual urine. Br J Urol 1979;51:129–34.

19. McGuire E, Woodside J, Borden T, et al. Prognostic value of urodynamic testing in myelodysplastic patients. J Urol 1981;126:205.

20. Bump R, Coats K, Cundiff G, et al. Diagnosing intrinsic sphincter deficiency: urethral closure pressure, urethral axis, and Valsalva leak point pressures. Am J Obstet Gynecol 1997;177:303.

21. McGuire E, Fitzpatrick C, Wan J, et al. Clinical assessment of urethral sphincter function. J Urol 1993;150:700.

22. Lane T, Shah P. Leak-point pressures. BJU Int 2000;86:942–9.

23. Horbach NS, Ostegard DR. Predicting intrinsic sphincter dysfunction in women with stress incontinence. Obstet Gynecol 1994;84:188–92.

24. Ghoniem G, Elgamasy A, El Sergany R, et al. Grades of intrinsic sphincter deficiency associated with female stress urinary incontinence. Int Urogynecol J 2002;13:99–105.

Chapter 9

Cystoscopy

Alfred E Bent

Introduction

Visualization of bladder and urethra is important for a number of indications (Table 9.1). Most often this is performed in the office (clinic) setting with topical anesthesia.[1]

Instrumentation

Instrumentation includes the urethroscope, cystoscope, light source, infusing medium, video camera, and attachments for recording images in video or still format.[2,3]

Table 9.1 Indications for diagnostic cystoscopy and urethroscopy

Recurrent urinary tract infection

Irritative bladder and urethral symptoms

Hematuria

Urogenital fistula

Urethral or bladder diverticulum

Complicated urinary stress incontinence

Unresolved overactive bladder

Suspected interstitial cystitis

Calculus

Suspected bladder or urethral cancer

Obstructive voiding symptoms

Suspected foreign body

Assessment of ureteral function (especially postoperative)

Staging for cervical cancer

The urethroscope consists of an external sheath (sizes 15 and 24 Fr) and a 0° lens. The larger sheath can be used in most patients and affords rapid infusion of liquid medium, usually water. The smaller sheath provides almost no flow of infusion liquid, but provides access to small-caliber urethras, as well as allowing vaginoscopy in pediatric patients (Figure 9.1).

The cystoscope (Figure 9.2) consists of a sheath (size 17–28 Fr), telescope (0°, 30°, 70°, and 120°), bridge to connect sheath and telescope, and the other equipment as for urethroscopy, including infusion medium, light source, camera, and image recorders. The 17 Fr sheath is used in most diagnostic work, though a 15° sheath is available for pediatric work. The 30° lens is adequate for most diagnostic studies, but the 70° telescope may be required in the presence of elevation of the urethrovesical junction, such as after colposuspension procedures, and is a must for the operating room.[4] The telescopes have a field marker, a blackened notch, on the outside of the visual field opposite the angle of the deflection (opposite the light cord post), which helps facilitate orientation. The distal end of the cystoscope

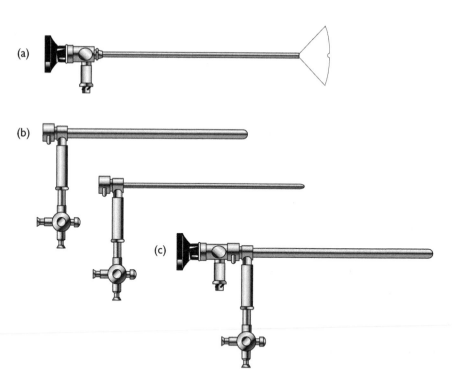

Figure 9.1 Components of the urethroscope: (a) telescope; (b) sheaths; (c) urethroscope. (Reproduced with permission from Cundiff GW, Bent AE. Endoscopic Diagnosis of the Female Lower Urinary Tract. London: WB Saunders, 1999:13.)

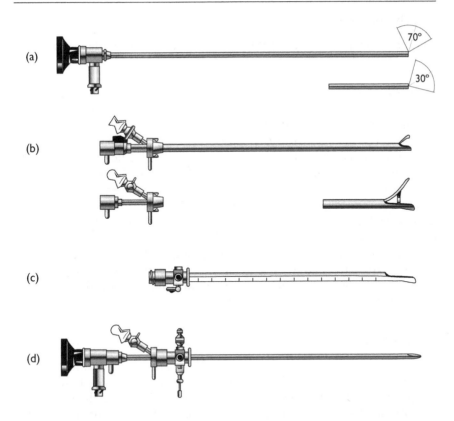

Figure 9.2 Components of the cystoscope: (a) telescopes; (b) bridges; (c) sheath; (d) rigid cystoscope. (Reproduced with permission from Cundiff GW, Bent AE. Endoscopic diagnosis of the female lower urinary tract. London: WB Saunders, 1999:10.)

sheath is fenestrated to permit use of instrumentation in the angled field of view. It is also beveled, opposite the fenestra, to increase the comfort of the introduction of the cystoscope into the urethra. The bridge allows instrumentation with a grasper, biopsy instruments, scissors, or ureteral catheters, and this may be aided by an Albarran bridge that has a deflector mechanism at the end of the inner sheath. Unlike the rigid cystoscope, the flexible cystoscope combines the optical systems and irrigation-working channel in a single unit. The coated tip is 15–18 Fr in diameter and 6–7 cm in length; the working unit makes up half the length. The flexibility of the fibers permits incorporation of a distal tip-deflecting mechanism, controlled by a lever at the eyepiece that will deflect the tip 290° in a single plane.

Urethroscopy

The urethroscope is placed at the urethral meatus with sterile water infusing rapidly, and the instrument is passed slowly through the urethra toward the bladder neck, while maintaining the urethra in the center of the field. The urethral mucosa is pink, and may show gland openings, as well as longitudinal folds (Figure 9.3). The urethrovesical junction (bladder neck) is passed as the scope enters the bladder. Fronds, polyps, and cysts are a normal variant at the bladder neck (Figure 9.4). With the bladder partly filled, maneuvers are conducted at the bladder neck that include the commands 'hold your urine', 'squeeze your rectum', 'strain down', and 'cough'. The most important observations are that the bladder neck moves with these procedures, and during the hold maneuvers it will close (Figure 9.5). A scarred bladder neck will appear pale and will have little movement with strain or cough (Figure 9.6). The urethra is then palpated while the urethroscope is withdrawn over the palpating finger. This may elicit excretion of mucus from the periurethral glands, or can express pus from a suburethral diverticulum. A fistula between urethra and vagina will be obvious, and a large one can reveal an examining glove.

Cystoscopy

Cystoscopy is performed by lubricating the sheath with lidocaine 2% gel, starting the infusion of sterile water, and placing the cystoscope (fenestrated end pointing up) into the urethra while advancing it toward the umbilicus. The bladder bubble appears as a landmark at the dome of the bladder

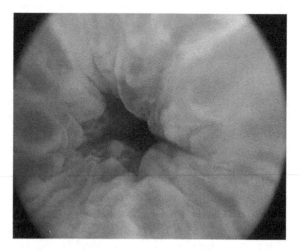

Figure 9.3 Normal urethral mucosa. (See also color image on p. xxiv)

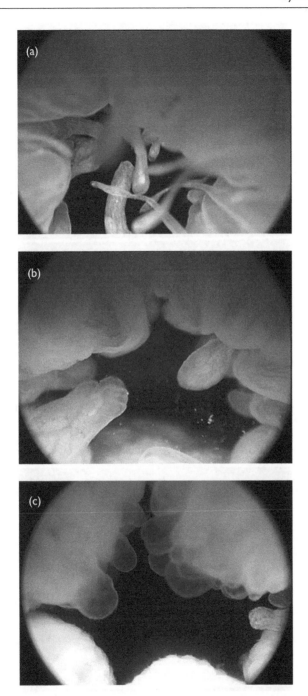

Figure 9.4 (a) Fronds, (b) polyps, and (c) cysts at the bladder neck. (See also color image on p. xxv)

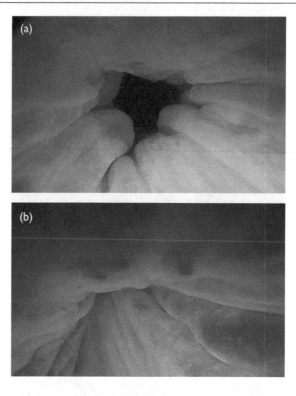

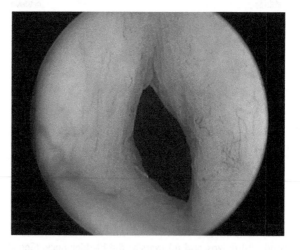

Figure 9.5 Maneuvers at bladder neck: (a) bladder neck open and (b) bladder neck closed. (See also color image on p. xxvi)

Figure 9.6 Scarred bladder neck. (See also color image on p. xxvi)

(Figure 9.7). Examination of the bladder proceeds in clockwise fashion as each hour is examined from 1 to 5, 11 to 7, and then 6 to 8 over the trigone and ureteral openings. The angle of view is 180° opposite the light post on the telescope. Examination is aided by moving the cystoscope downward and to the patient's right leg to observe the left upper area of the bladder (1 to 3 o'clock). Elevating the cystoscope will allow observation of the trigone and ureters. A vaginal finger may have to be placed to elevate the trigone or prolapsed anterior vaginal wall in order to view the trigonal area.

The bladder wall should appear pink with a light background of vasculature (Figure 9.7). The trigone may have a granulated appearance, and the ureters are located at the lateral margin of the trigone (Figure 9.8). Inflammatory mucosal abnormalities will appear as red dots or blotches (Figure 9.9). Surface cysts are common at the trigone, and are known as cystitis cystica (Figure 9.10). Trabeculation is the prominent pattern of ridges observed in the muscle of the bladder wall, sometimes as a result of outlet obstruction, or sometimes just with normal aging (Figure 9.11). Foreign bodies are an obvious abnormality (Figure 9.12). Bladder tumors take on a number of appearances, including papillary projections, smooth folds above the bladder surface, and obvious projections of abnormal tissue (Figure 9.13). The bladder should readily fill with 250 ml of fluid, and at the end of observation can be filled to 350–500 ml to determine bladder capacity. This amount is recorded on the dictated report.

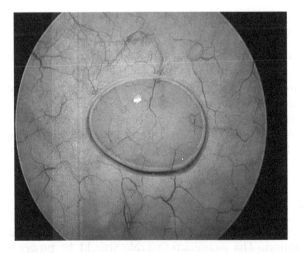

Figure 9.7 Normal bladder wall. (See also color image on p. xxvii)

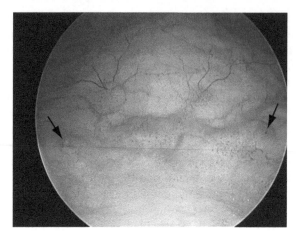

Figure 9.8 Bladder trigone (arrows mark ureteral orifices). (See also color image on p. xxvii)

Preparation and aftercare

The procedure is performed as a no-touch technique, and sterile draping is not required. The urethral meatus is cleansed with an antiseptic solution prior to the procedure. Instruments need regular cleaning and sterilization according to each facility's guidelines. Antibiotic prophylaxis after cystoscopy is not mandatory, though if used it may be better utilized as a preoperative dose.[5] Some patients have urethral discomfort after the procedure and phenazopyridine may be used every few hours for 24 hours.

Cystoscopy during pelvic reconstructive surgery

Operative cystoscopy requires the 70° lens for observation of the entire bladder after difficult gynecologic surgery, pelvic floor surgery, or incontinence procedures. When examining for ureteral patency, 2.5–5 ml of indigo carmine is injected intravenously, and the dye will appear at the ureteral openings after 6–7 minutes. The 30° lens along with Albarran bridge will be required if ureteral catheters need to be passed. It remains useful to perform these procedures with video for ease of examination and maneuvering.

Summary

Office cystoscopy may be performed readily on an outpatient basis without need for sedation. The examination table should be power-regulated to move patients easily from a sitting position to the appropriate examination

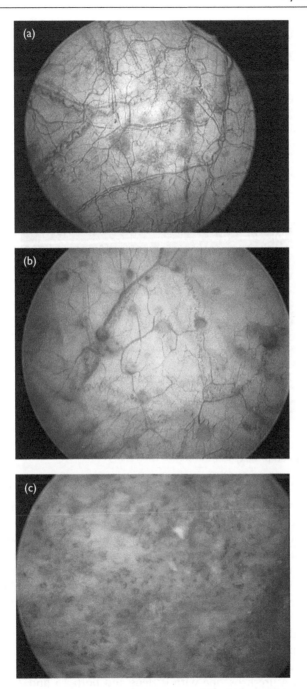

Figure 9.9 Abnormal mucosal surface of bladder: (a) spots of inflammation, (b) inflamed bladder wall, and (c) extensive inflammation of bladder wall. (See also color image on p. xxviii)

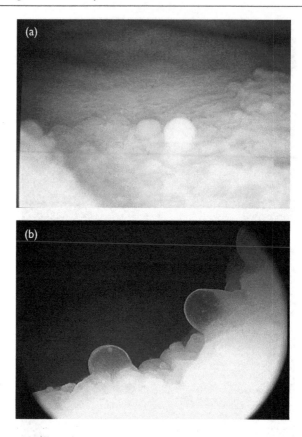

Figure 9.10 Cystitis cystica at trigone: (a) opaque and yellow cysts and (b) clear cysts. (See also color image on p. xxix)

position. The table can also be used for other examinations. The room will require a sink for cleaning instruments and a space for cold sterilization. A bathroom and change area should be adjacent to the room. Video equipment and image capture are essential for recording appropriate images and allowing examination while the examiner sits comfortably and maneuvers the telescope with attached video. The light source must be of high quality and power, and the light cable of 6 feet or less and optimally functioning. The infusion medium of water may be suspended on an intravenous pole and a normal intravenous infusion set used to deliver the fluid through the scope. A pressure bag is not required. A hysteroscope with 30° lens can be used to evaluate most female bladders, allowing use of only one instrument. Ideally, a urethroscope with 0° lens and both 15 and 24 Fr sheaths will allow appropriate examination of the urethra, or can be used as a vaginoscope even in the pediatric age group. Cystoscopy is ideally

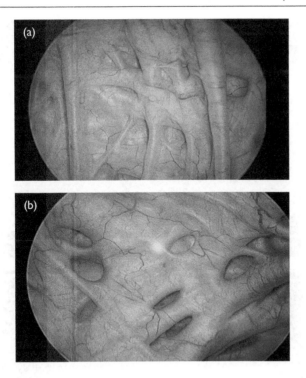

Figure 9.11 Trabeculated bladder muscle: (a) moderately severe and (b) severe with cellules. (See also color image on p. xxx)

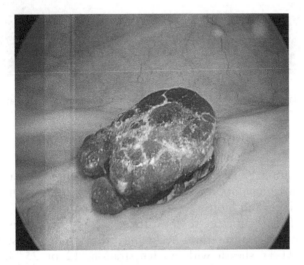

Figure 9.12 Bladder stone. (See also color image on p. xxx)

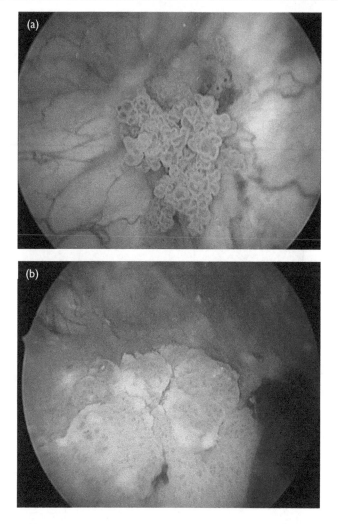

Figure 9.13 Bladder tumors: (a) papillary transitional cell type and (b) flat invasive type. (See also color image on p. xxxi)

performed with a 17 Fr sheath and 70° lens. For office operative manipulation, the instrumentation would include a 22 Fr sheath with 30° lens, an Albarran bridge, and biopsy forceps, scissors, and grasper. This is seldom required in female office cystoscopy. If periurethral bulking is done in the office using the transurethral technique, the required instrumentation includes a 21 Fr sheath with no fenestration, 12 or 25° lens, and an operative needle and needle guide.

References

1. Cundiff GW, Bent AE. The contribution of urethrocystoscopy to evaluation of lower urinary tract dysfunction. Int Urogynecol J 1996;7:307–11.
2. Cundiff GW, Bent AE. Endoscopic diagnosis of the female lower urinary tract. London: WB Saunders, 1999.
3. Cundiff GW, Bent AE. Cystourethroscopy. In: Baggish MS, Karram MM, eds. Atlas of Pelvic Anatomy and Gynecologic Surgery. London: WB Saunders, 2001: 721–46.
4. McLennan MT, Bent AE. Incidental cystotomy during obstetrical and gynecological surgery. J Pelvic Surg 1997;3:260–3.
5. Cundiff GW, McLennan MT, Bent AE. Randomized trial of antibiotic prophylaxis for combined urodynamics and cystourethroscopy. Obstet Gynecol 1999;93:749–52.

References

Chapter 10

Imaging

Nirit Rosenblum

Introduction

The evaluation of pelvic floor disorders, including incontinence of urine or feces, pelvic organ prolapse, voiding dysfunction, pain syndromes, and sexual dysfunction, depends on a thorough history and detailed physical examination as well as accurate, objective information obtained by imaging of the pelvis and its contents. Historically, imaging techniques in both gynecology and urology have relied upon noninvasive modalities such as transabdominal and transvaginal ultrasound or more invasive modalities such as defecography, endoanal ultrasound, and cystography (Table 10.1). Each of these techniques boasts its diagnostic advantages; however, none provides comprehensive information about pelvic and vaginal organ anatomy as well as dynamic function of the pelvic floor. The development of functional magnetic resonance imaging (MRI) directed at pelvic organ anatomy, pelvic organ prolapse, and pelvic floor function as a dynamic modality has revolutionized the evaluation and objective quantification of female pelvic disorders. Functional cine-MRI has become a well-accepted method of imaging both pelvic contents and pelvic floor function.[1] This chapter reviews the technique of functional pelvic MRI, indications for its use, current supporting literature, and future directions.

Functional magnetic resonance imaging of the pelvis

Magnetic resonance imaging has numerous advantages over standard radiography, ultrasound and computed tomography (CT) scanning in assessing pelvic organ pathology and pelvic floor function, including lack of radiation exposure, excellent quality of soft tissue contrast, multiplanar imaging, noninvasive modality, lack of exposure to nephrotoxic contrast material, and capability for dynamic evaluation with cine-loop sequences. Both static and dynamic phase images can be obtained to assess pelvic floor mobility and/or prolapse of the three vaginal compartments. Furthermore, MRI

Table 10.1 Imaging modalities for pelvic floor disorders

Imaging	Screening advantages
Noninvasive	
Transabdominal ultrasound	Uterine, adnexal pathology
	Bladder wall morphology
	Post-void residual urine
Transvaginal ultrasound	Uterine, adnexal pathology
	Cervical pathology
	Periurethral/vaginal wall pathology
	Vaginal wall vascularity
	Clitoral anatomy and vascularity
Dynamic cine-magnetic resonance imaging	Pelvic organ pathology
	Soft tissue pathology
	Urethral/periurethral pathology
	Intestinal pathology
	Sagittal two-dimensional anatomy
	Pelvic floor dynamic function:
	Pelvic organ prolapse
	Levator ani function
	Incontinence of urine/feces
	Perineal pathology
	Anal sphincter pathology/function
	Ureteral pathology
Invasive	
Defecography/evacuation proctography	Anal sphincter pathology and function
	Rectocele
	Intussusception and rectal prolapse
Endoanal ultrasound	Internal and external anal sphincter pathology
	Rectal mucosal pathology
Cystography	Cystocele
	Incontinence
	Bladder wall pathology
	Vesicoureteral reflux

can identify external anal sphincter defects perhaps more readily than endoanal ultrasound, because of the high degree of contrast between the anal sphincter and perirectal fat.[2] Excellent temporal resolution is attained through rapid sequence T2–weighted MRI, a relatively fast imaging modality with limited patient discomfort.

Dynamic pelvic MRI is a useful preoperative tool in assessing all three vaginal compartments for prolapse when planning surgical therapy. If physical examination findings are equivocal or do not necessarily correlate with

Table 10.2 Compartments of pelvic organ prolapse and pathology

Vaginal compartment	Anatomic defect
Anterior	Urethral hypermobility/incontinence Bladder neck hypermobility Cystocele
Apical/middle	Uterine prolapse Cervical elongation Enterocele/peritoneocele Sigmoidocele
Posterior	Rectocele Enterocele (rectovaginal septum) Rectal prolapse Perineal hernia/perineocele Anal sphincter defects

symptomatology, functional pelvic MRI can aid in the assessment of anterior, apical, and posterior compartment prolapse (Table 10.2). Perineal herniation or convexity can be detected during the dynamic phase, which may prompt perineal repair and perineal body reconstruction. Anal sphincter morphology can be assessed in cases of fecal incontinence or incontinence of flatus. In addition, hydroureter can be identified in cases of severe cystocele with ureteral traction/kinking. Abnormalities of the endometrium, uterine body, or adnexa may alter surgical management and necessitate hysterectomy and/or oophorectomy. Benign enlargement of the uterus, often caused by leiomyomatous tumors, can be accurately assessed in three dimensions and provide valuable information regarding the feasibility of a planned vaginal hysterectomy or prolapse repair.

Magnetic resonance imaging technique

Dynamic pelvic MRI protocols vary and can include vaginal or rectal contrast, static and dynamic phase images, multiplanar imaging in sagittal, coronal, and axial planes and endoanal coils for anal sphincter evaluation. In general, the bladder should be at least half full. A phased array coil is positioned low around the patient's pelvis. The static portion of the study is carried out in sagittal, coronal, and axial planes to include all three pelvic compartments. The dynamic phase includes both HASTE (half-Fourier acquisition single shot turbo spin echo) and FISP (Fast Imaging with Steady state Precession) sequences during graded degrees of pelvic straining (Valsalva maneuvers), which can be looped into a cine-MRI. The HASTE sequence is a series of single shots that maintains high spatial resolution through partial acquisition. The average total time of this acquisition is less than 2 minutes. The FISP sequence is a continuous method of image acquisition, which allows improved temporal resolution. Both sequences are often employed to assess pelvic floor mobility, function, and degree of prolapse. Dynamic MRI proctography can be carried out using rectal gel and image acquisition during rest, squeeze, and defecation.[3]

Prior to the functional cine-MRI study, there is no need for patient preparation. However, the patient should be familiarized with the protocol and the instructions for progressive straining maneuvers during the course of the examination. Some radiologists recommend opacification of the vagina and/or rectum using sonography gel for improved visualization of pelvic structures, such as the fornix of the vagina and the rectovaginal septum. This contrast gel is easily administered without significant patient discomfort, and is inexpensive and well tolerated.[2]

In general, the protocol for functional pelvic floor MRI is divided into static and dynamic pulse sequences. The static component includes T2-weighted turbo spin-echo sequences of the pelvis in both axial and sagittal orientations. These high-resolution, static images provide a morphologic assessment of pelvic structures, including the pelvic floor musculature. In addition, incidental anomalies or pathologic findings can be elucidated. The urethral complex as viewed in the axial plane serves as a point of reference for the dynamic sequence.

The dynamic sequence consists of a T2-weighted FISP or HASTE sequence, depending on the radiologist's preference. The sagittal images allow visualization of all three pelvic compartments at the same time, whereas the axial images provide valuable information about the urogenital hiatus and its contents, including the perineum. The patient is asked to relax the pelvic floor muscles, followed by slow contractions. Then, the patient is asked to progressively increase intra-abdominal pressure by straining, and in some cases by defecation. Additional coronal images can be performed to assess the levator ani muscles during straining. The total time of acquisition varies between 20 and 30 minutes.[2]

Magnetic resonance image analysis

The analysis of all static and dynamic images is relatively easy to perform and provides useful information for the clinician. Several reference lines have been proposed to assess the degree of pelvic floor relaxation and prolapse. The extent of pelvic organ prolapse is generally quantified in reference to three defined lines on the mid-sagittal image where maximal descent is visualized during the dynamic sequence:

• the pubococcygeal line (PCL) is a straight line between the inferior rim of the pubic bone and the last visible coccygeal joint (Figure 10.1)

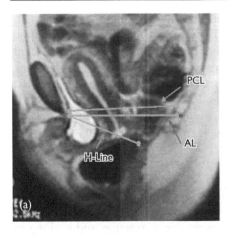

Normal

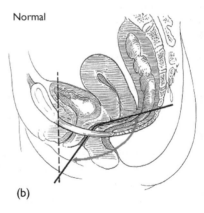

(b)

Figure 10.1 (a) Dynamic pelvic MRI during Valsalva maneuver in the sagittal plane with reference lines highlighted in red: PCL = pubococcygeal line, AL = axial line, H-line = hymenal line. (b) Schematic illustration of normal pelvic organ anatomy, with normal vaginal axis line depicted.

- the second line is the horizontal tangent of the inferior rim of the pubic bone (axial line; AL)
- and the third line is the hymenal line (HL) drawn through the long axis of the pubic bone on the mid-sagittal image.

The pelvis is generally divided into three anatomic compartments. A structure from within each compartment is defined and its position described with respect to one of the three aforementioned reference lines, the pubococcygeal line being the most common. The most validated reference line is the PCL. Simply put, the PCL is a practical reference line used to describe descent of key pelvic structures.

The primary anatomic structures within the anterior compartment are the urethra, bladder neck and bladder base. Within the superior compartment, the distal-most aspect of the cervix or posterior fornix is evaluated in relation to the reference line. Finally, the most caudal aspect of the anterior rectal wall is utilized from the posterior compartment.[1]

Dynamic pelvic magnetic resonance imaging: compartmental prolapse

Anterior compartment prolapse

The anterior pelvic compartment assessed with dynamic pelvic MRI includes the urethra, bladder neck, and bladder. Stress urinary incontinence with associated bladder neck and/or urethral hypermobility can be visualized during Valsalva maneuvers on T2-weighted images. Bright-colored fluid can be visualized within the urethral lumen or vaginal vault consistent with urinary incontinence. The mobility of the urethra and bladder neck can be well-visualized during the dynamic or cine-portion of the MRI viewed in the mid-sagittal plane (Figure 10.2). Separation of the proximal urethra and bladder neck from the pubic symphysis, with associated hypermobility and posterior rotation, is well visualized on the sagittal images.

The degree of cystocele, including both central and lateral defects, is also well visualized with dynamic pelvic MRI (Figure 10.3). Bladder wall thickening can also be assessed in cases of severe bladder outlet obstruction. Furthermore, dilation of the ureters (hydroureter) can be incidentally discovered in association with severe cystocele due to traction and kinking of the ureters.

Superior/apical/middle compartment prolapse

Physical examination alone is often inadequate in assessing the degree of apical compartment prolapse. The degree of uterine descent during Valsalva maneuvers is difficult to appreciate when obscuring anterior or posterior compartment prolapse is present. In addition, cervical elongation, commonly seen in multiparous women, can cause confusion and be mistaken for uterine prolapse. Dynamic pelvic MRI is especially useful in assessing

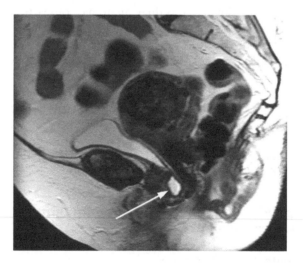

Figure 10.2 Dynamic pelvic MRI during Valsalva maneuver in the sagittal plane with incontinence demonstrated as bright fluid exterior to the urethra (arrow). Also noted is descent of the bladder neck with separation from the pubic symphysis.

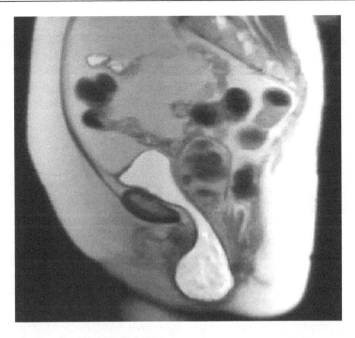

Figure 10.3 Dynamic pelvic MRI during Valsalva maneuver in the sagittal plane with severe cystocele visualized outside of the patient's introitus (grade IV).

the apical compartment (Figure 10.4). Pathology of the uterus can be uncovered (i.e. fibroids, uterine enlargement) and may alter surgical management. Cervical elongation can readily be distinguished from significant uterine prolapse. In cases of post-hysterectomy prolapse, the contents of the vault prolapse can be better defined. Enterocele, also termed peritoneocele, can be distinguished from cystocele as well as sigmoidocele (Figure 10.5). With both enterocele and peritoneocele, small intestinal contents, fat and fluid, are visualized within the herniating sac extending below the PCL.

Posterior compartment prolapse

Evaluation of the posterior compartment with dynamic pelvic MRI can assess for the presence of a rectocele, with defects in the rectovaginal septum, rectal prolapse, rectal or sigmoid intussusception, as well as anorectal junction descent. Rectocele is defined as a bulging and descent of the anterior rectal wall during straining maneuvers (Figure 10.6). This is readily identified on dynamic MRI in the sagittal plane as a gas-filled structure bulging below the PCL or even outside the introitus. Posterior herniation of the small intestine and other intra-abdominal contents (i.e. peritoneal fat,

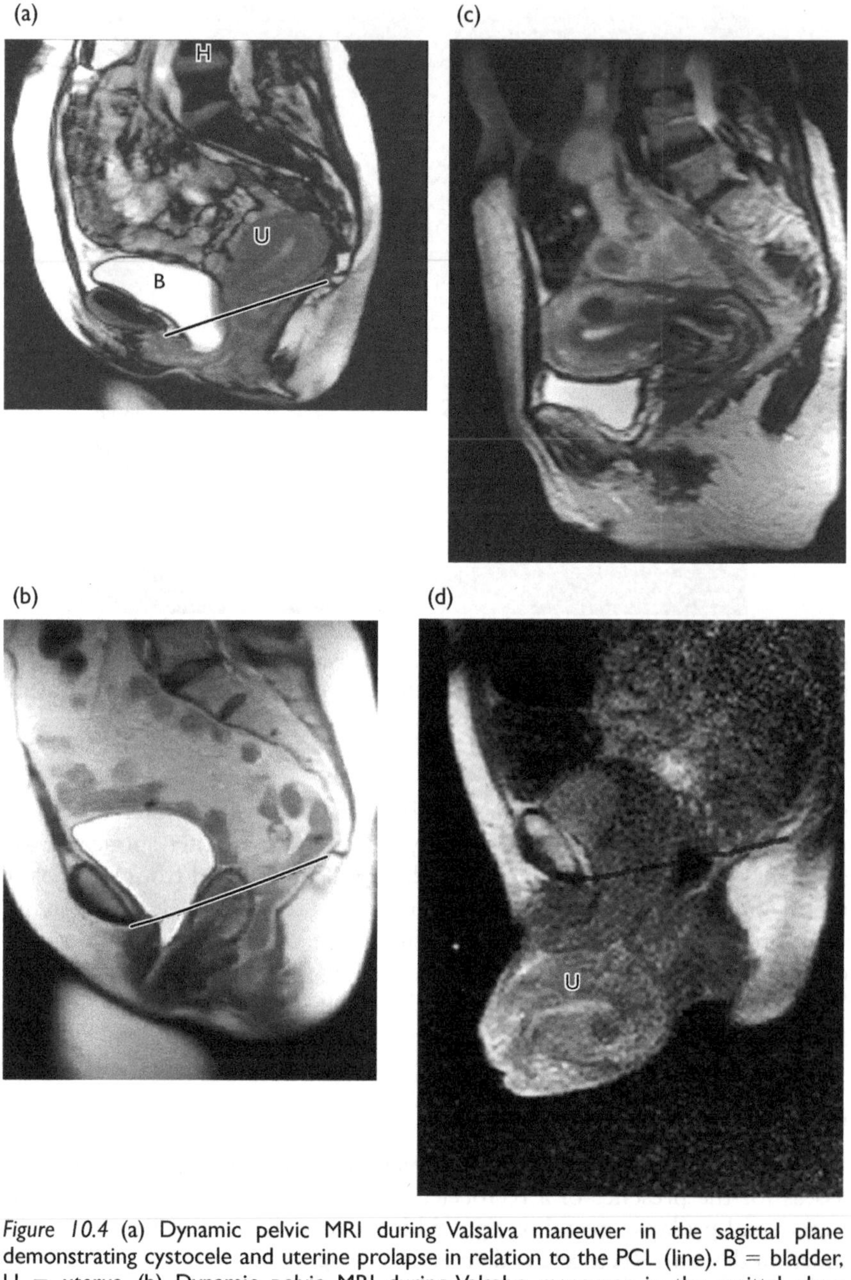

(a)

(c)

(b)

(d)

Figure 10.4 (a) Dynamic pelvic MRI during Valsalva maneuver in the sagittal plane demonstrating cystocele and uterine prolapse in relation to the PCL (line). B = bladder, U = uterus. (b) Dynamic pelvic MRI during Valsalva maneuver in the sagittal plane demonstrating uterovaginal prolapse in relation to the PCL (line). (c) Dynamic pelvic MRI at rest in the sagittal plane with uterus in normal anatomic orientation, well above the PCL, and (d) during Valsalva maneuver revealing complete uterine prolapse (eversion) outside of the introitus. U = uterus.

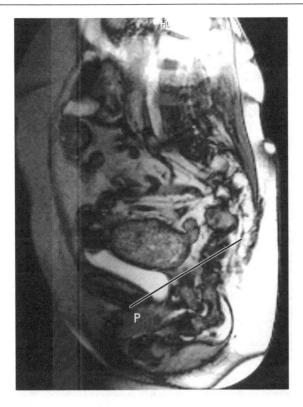

Figure 10.5 Dynamic pelvic MRI during Valsalva maneuver in the sagittal plane demonstrating large peritoneocele extending several centimeters below the PCL (line).

omentum) into the rectovaginal septum can be identified as a posterior enterocele or peritoneocele, where loops of bowel are visualized interposed between the vagina and rectum (Figures 10.7 and 10.8). Rectal prolapse can be identified as protrusion of the rectum, either partially or completely, through the anal orifice. Rectal intussusception is identified as rectal invagination which descends towards the anal canal, but does not extend through it. Descent of the anorectal junction is an indication of generalized pelvic floor relaxation.

Dynamic magnetic resonance imaging of defecatory disorders

Dynamic pelvic MRI is a minimally invasive imaging modality that can be utilized in the evaluation of both fecal incontinence and obstructed defecation. Fletcher et al compared dynamic pelvic MRI with endoanal ultrasound in

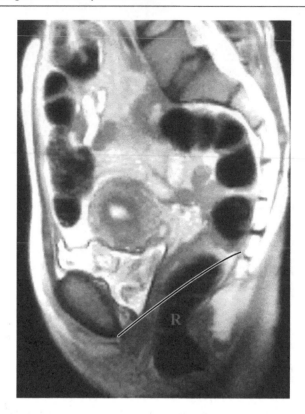

Figure 10.6 Dynamic pelvic MRI during Valsalva maneuver in the sagittal plane demonstrating large rectocele filled with gas (black) extending below the PCL.

assessing defects of the internal and external anal sphincters and found comparable results.[3] An endorectal coil is utilized followed by endoanal gel during evacuation. MRI was capable of identifying excessive perineal descent during straining and defecation as well as thinning or tears in the anal sphincter.

Fuchsjager et al describe the use of endoanal MRI in the evaluation of fecal incontinence.[4] MRI offers the distinct advantages of multiplanar imaging and high soft tissue contrast, which is especially useful in identifying discrete components of the external anal sphincter. A sphincter defect is identified as a discontinuity of the muscle ring, whereas scarring is defined as a hypointense deformation of the normal muscle layer pattern.

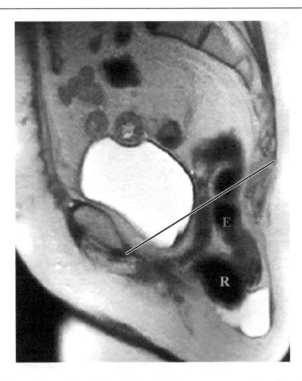

Figure 10.7 Dynamic pelvic MRI during Valsalva maneuver in the sagittal plane demonstrating posterior enterocele between the posterior vaginal wall and rectum. E = enterocele, R = rectocele.

Magnetic resonance imaging of levator ani morphology

Several authors have described the use of dynamic pelvic MRI in the evaluation of pelvic floor muscle morphology, function, and defects following vaginal delivery. Singh et al studied women with varying degrees of pelvic prolapse with three-dimensional pelvic MRI and assessed the following characteristics of the puborectalis muscle group: levator symphysis gap, the width of the levator hiatus, and the length of the levator hiatus.[5] These authors found that alterations in levator ani morphology did not necessarily correlate with the degree of prolapse. However, both the levator symphysis gap and the levator hiatus widen with increasing grades of prolapse.

Hoyte et al utilized magnetic resonance-based, three-dimensional color mapping to assess levator ani thickness variations in women, both symptomatic (stress incontinence or prolapse) and asymptomatic.[6] They found

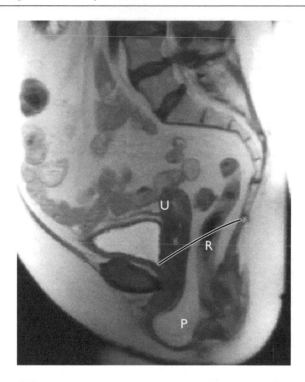

Figure 10.8 Dynamic pelvic MRI during Valsalva maneuver in the sagittal plane demonstrating posterior peritoneal contents herniating between the uterus and rectum. U = uterus, R = rectum, P = peritoneocele.

statistically significant differences in levator thickness and gaps amongst symptomatic versus asymptomatic women. This particular technique can help to further the understanding of pelvic floor dysfunction.

Conclusions

Dynamic pelvic magnetic resonance imaging is a noninvasive, safe, and accurate modality that is useful in assessing pelvic floor dysfunction, pelvic organ prolapse, defecatory disorders, pelvic pain syndromes, urinary and fecal incontinence, perineal descent and herniation, and reproductive organ pathology. Image analysis is reproducible and can be readily learned by clinicians without significant radiologic or MR experience. Furthermore, incidental pelvic organ pathology can be elucidated in a relatively accurate modality without the need for additional radiographic procedures.

References

1. Lienemann A, Sprenger D, Janben U, et al. Assesment of pelvic organ descent by use of functional cine-MRI: Which reference line should be used? Neurourol Urodyn 2004;23:33–7.
2. Lienemann A, Fischer T. Functional imaging of the pelvic floor. Eur J Radiol 2003;47:117–22.
3. Fletcher JG, Busse RF, Riederer SJ, et al. Magnetic resonance imaging of anatomic and dynamic defects of the pelvic floor in defecatory disorders. Am J Gastroenterol 2003;98:400–11.
4. Fuchsjager MH, Maier AG. Imaging fecal incontinence. Eur J Radiol 2003;47:108–16.
5. Singh K, Jakab M, Reid WM, et al. Three-dimensional magnetic resonance imaging assessment of levator ani morphologic features in different grades of prolapse. Am J Obstet Gynecol 2003;188: 910–15.
6. Hoyte L, Jakab M, Warfield SK, et al. Levator ani thickness variations in symptomatic and asymptomatic women using magnetic resonance-based 3-dimensional color mapping. Am J Obstet Gynecol 2004;191:856–61.

Chapter 11

Physiologic evaluation of the colon, rectum and anus

Jose Marcio N Jorge

Introduction

Colorectal physiologic testing will allow, in about 50–75% of cases, stratification of potentially disabling and highly prevalent disorders such as fecal incontinence and chronic idiopathic constipation into diverse causative diagnoses with distinctive therapeutic approaches.[1] The evaluation of these complex disorders will usually require a combination of studies and a multidisciplinary approach. Physiologic tests of practical value include anorectal manometry, colonic transit time study, videodefecography, electroneuromyography, and anal ultrasound.[2]

Indications for colorectal testing

Exclusion of both intestinal and systemic organic etiologies is imperative prior to referring the patient with functional symptoms to the physiology laboratory. Both barium enema and colonoscopy are comparable in the diagnosis of lesions associated with constipation; however, barium enema has the advantage of providing a permanent record, available for future evaluations, of the size, length, and anatomic abnormalities of the colon.

History and physical examination may dictate additional tests. In addition, a therapeutic schema is usually introduced, including dietary assessment, a diary of defecation, symptoms and, when indicated, psychologic evaluation. In constipated patients, supplemental fiber, increased fluid intake, and physical activity are helpful measures. This initial therapy will permit better evaluation of the severity of the symptom. Furthermore, symptoms may even improve, if they are dietary or psychologically related. Often, patients referred for colorectal physiologic testing present with refractory and severe idiopathic symptoms, and a combination of studies is usually indicated due to the complex etiology of these functional disorders.

Anorectal manometry

Anorectal manometry is an objective method of studying the physiologic apparatus of defecation provided by the anal sphincter. Manometric sensing devices include microballoons, microtransducers, and water-perfused catheters. Plastic multichannel catheters, perfused with water by a microperfusion system, are the most commonly used sensing devices, and measure the resistance by sphincters in terms of pressure to a constant flow of water through the port. A constant perfusion rate, usually 0.3 ml/channel/min is required to adequately measure the outflow from the tube. The most important advantage of perfused catheters is that multiple channels, more commonly 4–8 channels, can be set on a single catheter. Conventional anorectal manometry, using an intrarectal balloon, enables measurement of both resting and squeeze pressures, as well as the high pressure zone or functional anal canal length. Adjunct studies include assessment of rectoanal inhibitory reflex, rectal sensory threshold, rectal capacity, and rectal compliance.

The mean **anal canal resting tone** in healthy adults is generally in the range of 50–70mmHg, usually lower in women and in the elderly.[3] In the composition of the resting tone, the internal anal sphincter (IAS) is responsible for 50–85%, the external anal sphincter (EAS) accounts for 25–30%, and the remaining 15% is attributed to expansion of the anal cushions.[4] Because of both intrinsic myogenic and extrinsic autonomic neurogenic properties, the IAS is in a state of continuous maximum contraction and, therefore, forms a natural barrier to the involuntary loss of stool. A gradual increase in pressure is noted from proximal to distal in the anal canal; the highest resting pressures are usually recorded 1–2 cm cephalad to the anal verge. This *high-pressure zone* or *functional anal canal length*, which corresponds anatomically to the condensation of the smooth muscle fibers of the IAS, is shorter in women (2.0–3.0 cm) than in men (2.5–3.5 cm). The anal canal is also relatively asymmetric on its radial profile. The normal values for the *radial asymmetry index* are ≤ 10%; however, these values are subject to the technique and equipment used.[3]

During **maximal voluntary contraction or squeeze efforts**, the activity of the EAS and the pelvic floor muscles will increase intra-anal pressures to two or three times their baseline resting tone (100–180mmHg). However, due to muscular fatigue, maximal voluntary contraction of the EAS and levator ani can be sustained for only 40–60 seconds (Figure 11.1). In some patients, despite an initial normal squeeze pressure, a rapid decrease in values can be noted, and therefore, this inability of sustaining the voluntary contraction may represent either an initial or different mechanism of lesion. The *fatigue rate index* is a calculated measure (in minutes) of the time necessary for the sphincter to be completely fatigued to a pressure equivalent to the resting tone. According to Marcello et al,[5] the mean fatigue rate index is 3.3 minutes for volunteers, 2.8 minutes for constipated patients,

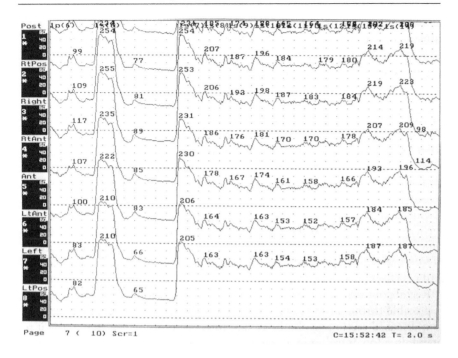

Figure 11.1 Voluntary contraction pressures of the anal canal, with assessment of the sphincter fatigue undex.

2.3 minutes for patients with seepage, and 1.5 minutes for incontinent patients. Unlike other skeletal muscles, which are usually inactive at rest, EAS and levator ani muscles have a predominance of type I fibers, which is characteristic of skeletal muscles of tonic contractile activity. Additionally, in response to conditions of threatened continence, such as increased intra-abdominal pressures and rectal distention, the EAS and PR reflexively or voluntarily contract further in order to prevent fecal leakage.

The **rectoanal inhibitory reflex** (RAIR), transient EAS contraction and pronounced IAS reflex relaxation in response to rectal distention, enables rectal contents to come into contact with the highly sensitive epithelial lining of the upper anal canal. By providing accurate distinction between flatus and feces, this 'sampling' mechanism is thought to have a role in the fine adjustment of anal continence. Although the IAS relaxes in response to rectal distention, it gradually reacquires its tone as the rectum accommodates to the distention. The RAIR is probably located entirely within the bowel wall; it is dependent upon mechanoreceptors in the rectum and independent of higher neural centers. When both reduced anal sensation and defective sampling mechanism occur, the patient may be completely unaware of impending incontinence. Absence of the RAIR in a patient with constipation is suggestive of Hirschsprung's disease, or in prevalent areas, of Chagas' disease.[6]

During manometry, **rectal sensory threshold** is evaluated by injecting progressive volume of air into an intrarectal balloon: normally with 10–40 ml of volume, patients will sense the balloon. The poor discriminatory quality of rectal sensation is probably due to the absence of sensory nerve endings in the rectum; these proprioceptors are more likely situated in adjacent pelvic structures, such as the levators, puborectalis, and anal sphincters. Diseases such as altered mental conditions (encephalopathy, dementia, and stroke) and sensory neuropathy (diabetes) may selectively reduce conscious sensation and awareness of rectal fullness. Although these patients may not recognize or respond to threats to continence, the autonomic pathways that mediate the RAIR may be intact. A fecal bolus in the rectum results in reflexive relaxation of the IAS. In these patients, that relaxation occurs before a sensation of rectal distention, which results in both fecal impaction and overflow incontinence.

Rectal contents must be accommodated if defecation is to be delayed; this is possible through the mechanisms of **rectal capacity** and **compliance**. The non-diseased rectum has both viscous and elastic properties that allow it to maintain a low intraluminal pressure while being filled, in order to preserve continence. Whether poor rectal compliance is a cause or a consequence of fecal incontinence is controversial. The fact that rectal compliance is frequently impaired in both idiopathic and traumatic incontinence suggests that decreased rectal compliance is rather a consequence of an incompetent anal sphincter. On the other hand, if rectal compliance deteriorates, smaller volumes of feces will result in higher intraluminal pressures causing urgency and incontinence.

Anorectal manometry is the most commonly used test in an anorectal physiology laboratory, especially in anal incontinence, in order to document the degree of sphincter impairment. Evaluation of anorectal pressure parameters is also helpful prior to operations of the colon, rectum, and anus, whenever the continence mechanism is endangered, due to the nature of the procedure or to an occult pre-existent sphincter lesion. In fact, occult, subclinical incontinence may be diagnosed only during physiologic testing, particularly during manometry. Anal manometry is often of no 'diagnostic value' in idiopathic constipation in adults, except in the rare cases of segmental Hirschsprung's disease. In these cases, more often in children and adolescents with constipation and encopresis, the absence of the RAIR should be correlated with rectal biopsy. In constipation, anal manometry provides supportive data for pelvic floor dysfunction: for example, high resting tone with an elongated functional anal canal and little voluntary augmentation suggests paradoxical puborectalis contraction. In addition, high rectal capacity and compliance may suggest outlet obstruction.

Colonic transit times

Colonic motility studies such as manometry or electromyography are of limited use due to the relative inaccessibility of the proximal colon. In addition, colonic manipulation and dilatation may compromise the fidelity of manometric recordings. Although these studies have been proposed to discriminate dysmotility patterns, pathognomonic of underlying pathophysiologic processes, currently these tests have not achieved relevance in clinical practice.

The colon accounts for approximately 80–90% of the total digestive transit time.[7] Therefore, colonic transit time has been primarily evaluated as the total digestive transit through the elimination of markers in the feces. The simplest and most practical method of evaluating colonic transit requires ingestion of 24 radiopaque markers and quantification of these markers on abdominal radiographs.[8] Normal total intestinal transit time involves elimination of at least 80% of markers on the fifth day of study.[8] Subsequently, segmental colonic transit time study was proposed as the ideal assessment of colonic transit.[9] Rather than measuring the elimination or clearance of markers, the index of transit time of this method was the actual number of retained markers on each colonic segment. The spinal processes and imaginary lines from the fifth lumbar vertebra to the pelvic outlet have been used to recognize the three segments of the large bowel (right colon, left colon, and rectosigmoid) on the radiographs. The classical technique of measuring segmental transit time consisted of a single ingestion of 20 or 24 markers followed by serial radiographs taken at 24-hour intervals until total elimination of markers occurred. When using 24 markers, the sum of the retained markers in each colonic segment on the successive radiographs represents the value (in hours) for each segmental transit time. In order to reduce irradiation exposure and achieve more practicality, subsequent technical modifications included multiple ingestion of markers, rather than multiple radiographs, and the use of markers of different shapes. However, the technique involving two radiographs, taken on days 3 and 5 after a single day ingestion of 24 radiopaque markers, may suffice. Prior to testing, a digital examination and, if necessary, a simple abdominal radiograph, are indicated to insure that the colon is cleared of any contrast material from previous studies and that there is no fecal impaction in the rectum. The use of enemas, laxatives, or any other medication known to affect gastrointestinal motility should be discontinued for 3 days prior to ingestion of the markers until completion of the study. Patients are instructed to maintain their normal diet; however, supplemental fiber such as bran or psyllium can be helpful to exclude dietary causes. The study may be repeated if the patient reports that the frequency during the study is not representative of usual bowel habits.

In normal individuals, markers reach the cecum within 8 hours after their ingestion. The mean and maximal values for normal individuals for the total colonic transit time are 36 and 55 hours, respectively. The mean segmental transit times are 12, 14, and 11 hours for right colon, left colon, and rectosigmoid, respectively; the maximal values for the segmental transit times are 22, 34, and 27 hours for right colon, left colon, and rectosigmoid, respectively.[7,9] The mean value of normal total colonic transit time is about 32 hours for men and 41 hours for women. This difference is even greater when the right colon transit time is analyzed separately. However, age does not seem to affect total colonic transit times. In children, although the rectosigmoid transit time is more prolonged, the total colonic transit time is similar to the adult, probably due to the proportional reduction of segmental transit times for the right and left colons.[9]

Colonic transit time assessment is especially indicated in the evaluation of patients with chronic idiopathic constipation, as it converts an otherwise hopelessly subjective symptom to an objective part of the medical record. Segmental transit times can help to uncover causative diagnoses, by stratifying motility disorders into two main patterns: outlet obstruction and colonic inertia. Outlet obstruction is characterized when the stasis of markers is limited to the rectosigmoid (Figure 11.2). Association of other tests, particularly videodefecography and anorectal manometry, is of paramount importance to diagnose the causative disorder.

Colonic inertia is characterized by diffuse stasis of markers throughout the colon, usually more markedly in the right colon. This condition typically affects young women as a severe and incapacitating symptom. The **pathophysiology** of colonic inertia remains unclear. Lesions of the myenteric plexus have been demonstrated in patients with colonic inertia; these lesions can be either primary or related to chronic use of laxatives.[10] Colonic inertia can be also associated with other symptoms of visceral stasis, and a hypothesis of a systemic disorder has been proposed. Its treatment, however, has been less controversial; total colectomy with ileorectal anastomosis may alleviate symptoms in 80–96% of cases, yet careful patient selection is mandatory.[11] Selection criteria include reassessment of severity of symptoms (history, transit times, and response to trials of therapy with laxatives and prokinetics), exclusion of small bowel dysmotility (lactulose H_2 breath test), and exclusion of pelvic floor dysfunction. If dyspeptic symptoms such as nausea, vomiting, heartburn, and bloating are present, gastric emptying studies are indicated in order to exclude a generalized gastrointestinal stasis.

Several factors, including diet, physical activity, and psychologic and hormonal factors, may affect digestive transit time results; therefore, significant variation is expected. However, reproducibility seems to be best for patients with idiopathic constipation and worst for colonic inertia; therefore, consideration should be given to repeat colonic transit studies before colec-

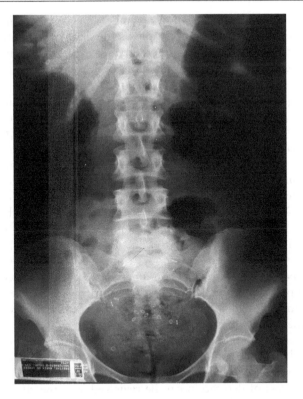

Figure 11.2 Colonic transit study on fifth day of study showing retention of markers in the rectosigmoid colon (outlet obstruction pattern).

tomy, in order to secure the diagnosis and improve outcome.[12] However, although proven useful, the value of the assessment of segmental transit times remains a controversial issue; accurate assessment still requires either multiple ingestion of markers or multiple abdominal radiographs.

Videodefecography

Standard anatomical examinations such as colonoscopy and barium enema detect essentially anatomic abnormalities, whereas functional disorders will require a radiographic study that demonstrates the physiologic process involved during rectal evacuation. Despite the apparent simplicity of the technique of defecography, defecation is a complex and somewhat poorly understood phenomenon, and both methodologic standardization and interpretation are still subjects of research. Specifically, defecography provides pelvic measurements at rest and during both squeeze and pushing, which are used to assess evacuation dynamics, anatomic detail, and rectal emptying. As a result, defecography allows the diagnosis of disorders such as paradoxical puborectalis contraction and excessive perineal descent syndromes, rectocele, intussusception, enterocele, and sigmoidocele.

The current patient preparation regimen for videodefecography includes a disposable phosphate enema 30 minutes prior to the procedure. With the patient initially placed in the left lateral decubitus position, a small amount (50 ml) of barium suspension is injected into the rectum in order to coat the rectal mucosa and enhance the contrast imagery, and a small amount of air is insufflated to outline the rectal mucosa. Subsequently, 250 ml (500 g) of a thick barium paste, assembled into a caulking gun to facilitate injection is introduced; less may be used if the patient experiences rectal fullness prior to that. The X-ray table is tilted upright to a 90° angle and the patient is comfortably seated on a water-filled radiolucent commode. In order to improve obtained imagery and reproduce normal physiology as closely as possible, a number of special commodes equipped with radiographic filters such as copper strips and water containers have been designed.[13] Lateral films of the pelvis can be taken at rest and during both squeeze and push for measurements. The patient is then asked to evacuate the rectal contents and, with the aid of fluoroscopy, the process of defecation is recorded on videotape. To study all phases of defecation effectively, the use of video recording is crucial in defecography, which is also known as cinedefecography, videodefecography, or videoproctography. By replaying the examination, the entire process of defecation can be reviewed, and the effects of abnormalities such as rectocele, intussusception, and nonrelaxing puborectalis in rectal emptying can be better evaluated, not only by the investigator, but also by the referring physician.

Technical variants have been proposed in an attempt to enhance the diagnostic capability of defecography, specifically to assist delineation of deep cul-de-sac pouches, enterocele, and sigmoidocele. Oral ingestion of 150 ml of barium contrast 1–3 hours prior to the examination may assist in the delineation of pelvic small bowel loops. The use of a tampon soaked in an iodine contrast medium placed in the posterior fornix of the vagina, either as an isolated method or combined with a voiding cystography (colpocysto-defecography), also helps to assess the depth of the rectogenital fossa and the eventual interposition of intra-abdominal content between the rectum and vagina. Dynamic anorectal endosonography has been recently proposed to evaluate enterocele during evacuation by measuring the change in the peritoneal–anal distance;[14] however, further studies are needed to prove its sensitivity for screening of this disorder. Dynamic pelvic resonance has also been proposed to investigate complex pelvic disorders, particularly in the diagnosis of cul-de-sac hernias and their contents, but despite an approximately 10-fold increase in cost, dynamic pelvic resonance imaging does not seem to have any significant advantage over videodefecography.[15]

Essentially, static proctography has been used to measure anorectal angle, perineal descent, and puborectalis length. The **anorectal angle** (ARA), better defined as the angle between the axis of the anal canal and the distal half of the posterior rectal wall, is the most quoted measurement on defecography.[13] The ARA is thought to be the result of the anatomic configuration of the U-shaped sling of puborectalis muscle around the anorectal junction. The resting ARA ranges from 70 to 140°, with mean of 92–114°. During evacuation, this angle becomes more obtuse, (110–180°), and more acute during squeeze (range 75–90°). **Perineal descent** is quantitatively defined by measuring the vertical distance between the position of the ARA and a fixed plane from the levator ani muscle to the pelvis, represented by the pubococcygeal line. The normal pelvic floor position is up to 1.8 cm below the pubococcygeal line at rest and up to 3 cm below the pubococcygeal line during maximal push effort; therefore, abnormally increased perineal descent has been classically defined as descent of more than 3 cm during evacuation compared with the value measured at rest. The **puborectalis length** is measured as the distance between the ARA and the pubic symphysis. The resting puborectalis length ranges from 14 to 16 cm. During squeeze, the puborectalis length is shorter (12–15 cm), and during evacuation, the muscle length increases (15–18 cm). Comparison of these measurements, along with the ARA, corroborates with the diagnosis of paradoxical puborectalis syndrome. However, wide ranges of normal values for each of these parameters are observed, and the exact value of any of these isolated parameters is of relatively little consequence. Instead, the role of static proctography is to provide a basis for relative comparison among resting, squeezing, and pushing values in a single patient.

Causative or associated 'anatomic' abnormalities, such as nonrelaxing puborectalis (puborectalis indentation), rectocele, internal rectal prolapse, sigmoidocele, and enterocele, can all be diagnosed by defecography. These findings, particularly a small rectocele and an intussusception, may be found in 25–77% of asymptomatic individuals.[13,16] Failure to recognize these variants of normal can easily lead to overdiagnosis and overtreatment. Therefore, a treatment decision should be made based upon both clinical history and evaluation of rectal emptying during videodefecography. During defecography, most individuals evacuate their rectum within 15–20 seconds; factors affecting rectal emptying rate include consistency of contents and patient embarrassment. Patients must be reassured and fully informed regarding the importance of the defecographic findings in their therapeutic approach.

Clinical applications

Defecography is particularly indicated in patients with chronic idiopathic constipation, to exclude causes of obstructed defecation. Additionally, in patients with idiopathic fecal incontinence, specifically when a history of chronic straining during evacuation is reported, defecography can be helpful to exclude internal rectal prolapse. Defecography can also help uncover causative disorders in patients with solitary rectal ulcer and chronic idiopathic rectal pain.

Nonrelaxing puborectalis syndrome

Nonrelaxing or paradoxical contraction puborectalis syndrome, also described as anismus or spastic pelvic floor, is a complex and poorly understood entity. It is characterized by paradoxical contraction, rather than relaxation, of the puborectalis and other striated pelvic floor muscles during attempted evacuation (Figure 11.3). The etiology of this dysfunction is obscure, but the behavioral disorder theory, based on uncoordinated relaxation of the striated anal sphincters during defecation, has been supported by a noticeable symptomatic improvement noted after biofeedback therapy.[17]

Although the exact incidence of nonrelaxing puborectalis syndrome remains unknown, it apparently represents an important etiologic factor in chronic idiopathic constipation. Typical clinical manifestations of non-relaxing puborectalis syndrome include symptoms of obstructed evacuation such as straining, tenesmus, and the sensation of incomplete evacuation as well as frequency of suppository or enema use or digitation. Physical examination may be suggestive of paradoxical contraction of the EAS and puborectalis muscle; however, patient embarrassment may cause a 'paradoxical

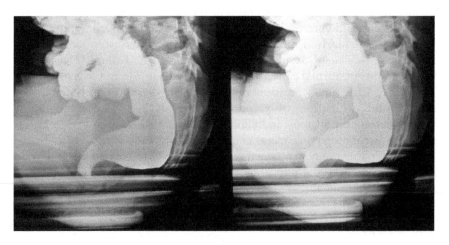

Figure 11.3 Paradoxical contraction puborectalis syndrome. Note an identical anorectal angle at rest and during push.

reaction'. Defecography and electromyography provide the best assessment of puborectalis muscle function. Electromyography assesses EAS and puborectalis neuromuscular activity, whereas cinedefecography allows measurement of the ARA, which is directly related to sphincter muscle activity. Defecographic criteria of nonrelaxing puborectalis syndrome include failure to open the ARA, persistence of the puborectalis impression during attempted defecation, an overly capacious rectum, a long and persistently closed anal canal, ballooning of the rectum, and the presence of compensatory anterior and posterior rectoceles. These findings can be associated with nonemptying, incomplete emptying, or even total evacuation after prolonged and difficult attempts.

Although useful, both defecography and electromyography have their own limitations. Voluntary contraction of the pelvic floor due to embarrassment may simulate a functional disorder on defecography. Likewise, the inability to relax the sphincter may occur during pushing as a response to fear or pain during the electromyographic assessment. Therefore, sensitivity, specificity, and predictive values of both electromyography and defecography are suboptimal, and the association of these tests may be necessary to permit optimal data accrual.[18] Nevertheless, defecography is probably superior, as it can detect associated abnormalities and demonstrate both dynamics of evacuation and rectal emptying. Although false-positive results may ensue due to the patient's fear of evacuating in front of others, the patient can be asked to evacuate in the privacy of a bathroom followed by fluoroscopic reassessment of the evacuated rectum.

Perineal descent syndrome

The perineal descent syndrome is the result of a vicious cycle involving excessive and repeated straining, protrusion of the anterior rectal wall into the anal canal, sensation of incomplete evacuation, weakness of the pelvic floor musculature, further straining, and ensuing progressive pelvic floor weakness. During defecography, increased dynamic perineal descent is considered when perineal descent exceeds values of 3 cm during a maximal push effort compared with values measured at rest.[13] Increased fixed perineal descent is described as perineal descent exceeding 4 cm at rest.

Excessive perineal descent is physical evidence that is indicative of pelvic floor weakness; however, it may merely represent one facet in a constellation of varied symptoms and findings. Patients with abnormally increased perineal descent may present with rectal prolapse, partial or major incontinence, obstructed evacuation, solitary rectal ulcer syndrome, or vague symptoms of incomplete evacuation or rectal pain.

Rectocele

Rectocele represents herniation of the rectal wall, with the anterior being much more common than the posterior. This condition is more prevalent in females, and factors such as multiparity and traumatic vaginal deliveries, which weaken the rectovaginal septum, are commonly implicated. The clinical history can be highly suspicious, as patients generally report either the need to press the posterior vaginal wall or rectal digitation in order to assist defecation. The presence of a rectocele can be assessed during physical examination by curving the examining finger and pressing it against the anterior rectal wall until it appears in the vagina, on the other side of the perineal body.

Prior to deciding a treatment option for a rectocele, it is crucial to assess both its clinical significance and concomitant functional disorders. Small rectoceles, less than 3 cm, can be found in up to 70% of asymptomatic women; however, rectoceles of greater diameter (>3 cm), with prolonged or even absent emptying, may very likely cause symptoms of constipation. However, the size of a rectocele as an isolated parameter does not seem to correlate with the severity of symptoms.[19] Common associated abnormalities include excessive perineal descent, enterocele, colonic inertia, and nonrelaxing puborectalis syndrome. Rectoceles can be found in up to 45% of patients with emptying disorders due to nonrelaxing puborectalis syndrome.[20] This type of rectocele usually represents a compensatory mechanism due to the functional closure of the anal canal during attempted defecation and consequently high intrarectal pressure. Under these circumstances, this finding is of primary importance, as biofeedback therapy rather than surgical treatment should be indicated.

Cul-de-sac hernias: enterocele and sigmoidocele

The cul-de-sac or pouch of Douglas can progressively extend caudally between the rectum and vagina and, in varying degrees, even as far as the perineum. Eventually, it progresses to become the site of a cul-de-sac or vaginal hernia. The hernia contents can include the omentum, small bowel and, occasionally, an elongated loop of sigmoid. Sigmoidocele, similar to an enterocele, is usually a component of a complex entity known as pelvic laxity or pelvic relaxation. This results from weakening of the supporting tissues of the vagina and pelvic diaphragm. Therefore, several defects may coexist, including excessive perineal descent, anterior rectocele, rectoanal intussusception or overt rectal prolapse, cystocele, or vaginal or uterine prolapse (Figure 11.4).

Enteroceles have been classified as primary when factors such as multiparity, advanced age, general lack of elasticity, obesity, constipation, or increased abdominal pressure are present; they are considered secondary following

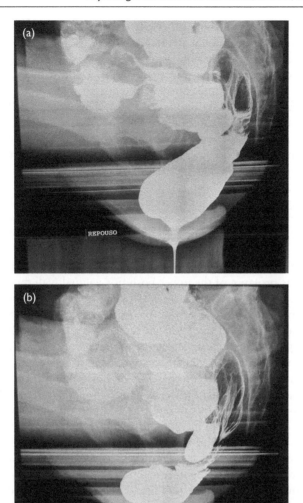

Figures 11.4 (a) and (b). During push (b), anterior rectocele, rectoanal intussusception, second-degree sigmoidocele, and excessive perineal descent are noted.

previous gynecologic procedures, specifically vaginal hysterectomies. The incidence of enterocele at 1 year or more following vaginal hysterectomy ranges from 6 to 25%; however, the incidence can be significantly reduced by suturing the uterosacral ligaments and obliterating the cul-de-sac.[21]

The pathophysiology of sigmoidocele in obstructed defecation is complex and several mechanisms may be involved, including collapse of the rectum, direct compression by the hernia contents, and stasis in the sigmoid. The contents of a cul-de-sac hernia split the fascia of Denonvilliers and weaken the rectovaginal septum. Consequently, the anterior rectal wall is exposed to the direct action of the abdominal pressure. Therefore, a collapse of the rectal ampulla, which is also influenced by factors such as the gradient of pressure and rate of flow, occurs during straining. In addition to a deep rectogenital pouch and slackening of the supporting structures of the uterus, intraoperative findings in these patients frequently include a long sigmoid loop and elongated proximal mesorectum. Unlike the small bowel, a herniated sigmoid is more prone to stasis due to the larger diameter and more solid contents. Consequently, symptoms of pelvic discomfort, sensation of incomplete evacuation, and prolonged straining can be more severe in patients with sigmoidocele.

Although a severe cul-de-sac hernia can be diagnosed during physical examination, as prolapse of the upper posterior vaginal wall during Valsalva maneuver, more accurate assessment of this entity, especially sigmoidocele, became possible only after the advent of defecography. Adequate technique to optimize the diagnosis of sigmoidocele on defecography includes the use of videorecording, systematic instillation of air and barium suspension, and injection of a substantial amount of barium paste. If necessary, the test may be performed 1–3 hours after ingestion of barium contrast medium to delineate small bowel loops. Other technical modifications recommended include the association of colpocystography and peritoneography.

In order to differentiate an incidental finding from a clinically significant sigmoidocele, a classification system has been proposed.[22] This classification is based on the degree of descent of the lowest portion of the sigmoid loop during maximum straining in relation to the following pelvic anatomic landmarks: pubis, coccyx, and ischium. First-degree sigmoidocele corresponds to an intrapelvic loop of sigmoid which does not surpass the pubococcygeal line, second-degree sigmoidocele is noted when the sigmoid loop is situated below the pubococcygeal line but remains above the ischiococcygeal line, and third-degree sigmoidocele is considered if the sigmoid loop transcends the ischiococcygeal line. This classification system yielded excellent correlation between the mean level of sigmoidocele, degree of sigmoid redundancy, and clinical symptoms.

Intussusception

Intrarectal and rectoanal intussusception represent initial phases of rectal prolapse: a fold develops in the rectal wall during push and prolapses into the rectum. Subsequently, the intussusception descends to obstruct the anal canal and finally becomes an external prolapse. As with rectocele, intussusception can represent either a mere defecographic finding or can be the cause of obstructed defecation. Criteria of clinical importance include the presence of transverse or oblique infolding of >3 mm of thickness, formed by invagination of the rectal wall, causing obstruction to rectal evacuation. These findings must be interpreted in light of the patient's clinical history. More advanced degrees of intussusception can cause rectal pain or even lead to solitary rectal ulcer syndrome, with discharge of blood or mucus through the rectum.

Electromyography

Anal electromyography (EMG) is the recording of myoelectrical activity from the striated sphincter at rest, during voluntary and reflex contraction, and simulated defecation. This study can be performed using needle, wire, or cutaneous patch electrodes. The concentric needle EMG has achieved more widespread acceptance in North America than other techniques. The sphincter muscle halves are independently examined both at rest and during squeezing, coughing, and attempted evacuation. A normal study is defined as the recruitment of an ample number of motor units with normal amplitude and duration while squeezing and coughing, and either electrical silence or a marked decrease in motor unit potentials during pushing.

Conventional concentric needle EMG is especially valuable in the assessment of fecal incontinence by providing quantification of motor unit potentials (MUPs), mapping EAS defects, and assessing reinnervation patterns (Figure 11.5). Decreased recruitment of MUPs is found in approximately 60% of patients with fecal incontinence, and polyphasic MUPs can be demonstrated in 40% of these patients.[23] Increased amplitude and duration of MUPs may also be demonstrated in injured areas. These findings are characteristic of injury, denervation, and subsequent partial reinnervation of the EAS and puborectalis from adjacent intact neuromuscular units.

Reinnervation, however, seems to be best assessed with single-fiber EMG, as extensive muscle atrophy results in insufficient MUPs to be evaluated with the concentric needle electrode. Single-fiber EMG allows calculation of fiber density, which is the mean number of single muscle fiber action potentials recorded within the electrode uptake area. Normally, at least four needle insertions are required with small adjustments of the position of the electrode during the recording process in order to calculate the mean number of single-fiber action potentials for 20 different positions within the muscle. The normal single-fiber EMG value for the EAS is 1.5 ± 0.16, and it increases with age and in incontinent patients. Although single-fiber EMG permits quantification of the injury, it does not alter clinical management any more than does concentric needle EMG. Moreover, single-fiber studies are more uncomfortable for the patient than are concentric needle examinations. Noninvasive surface or anal plug electrodes have also been

(a)

Esq Sphincter ani (Spont)

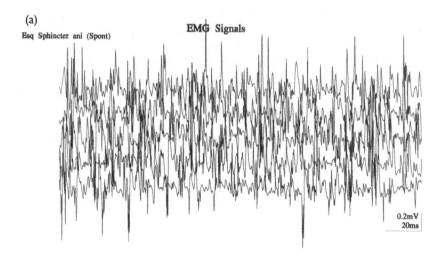

EMG Signals

0.2mV
20ms

(b)

Esq Sphincter ani (Spont)

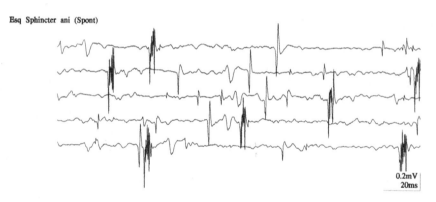

0.2mV
20ms

Figures 11.5 Electromyographic (EMG) tracings showing normal (a) and decreased recruitment of motor unit potentials (MUPs) along with polyphasic MUPs (b).

proposed; however, detailed findings of denervation and reinnervation are less likely to be demonstrated with these devices. In patients with idiopathic constipation, EMG may corroborate with the diagnosis of nonrelaxing puborectalis syndrome if doubt persists after defecography. Failure to achieve a significant decrease in the electrical activity of the EAS and puborectalis during attempted evacuation is considered as a criteria for the EMG diagnosis of nonrelaxing puborectalis syndrome. For this particular purpose, surface electrodes may be of use.

Pudendal nerve terminal motor latency

Pudendal nerve terminal motor latency (PNTML) measurement is a simple method of assessing pudendal nerve function. This test indicates the integrity of the distal motor innervation of the pelvic floor musculature. PNTML measurement is assessed transrectally with the patient placed in the left lateral decubitus position. The sensor consists of two stimulating electrodes located at the tip of the index finger of a glove and two surface recording electrodes incorporated into it. The ischial tuberosities are used as landmarks in the assessment of the pudendal nerves. Stimuli of 22 mV amplitude and 0.1 ms duration are applied to the nerves. These stimuli are given at 1 s intervals while the tip of the finger is gradually moved until the sphincter is felt to contract around the base of the finger and the motor unit action potential achieves a maximum amplitude. The latency from each stimulus to the evoked muscle action potential in the EAS is recorded on each side. The mean PNTML is calculated from the best amplitude measured. The normal value of PNTML is 2.0 ± 0.2 ms.[2] Latencies greater than 2.2 ms are considered excessive and representative of pudendal neuropathy (Figure 11.6).

PNTML is particularly important in suspected neurogenic incontinence and in parous women prior to sphincter repair. This test is the most important predictor of functional outcome after sphincter repair, as neuropathy, even when unilateral, is associated with poor postoperative functional results.[24] However, PNTML is not a quantitative method; it is a measurement of the fastest motor conduction in the pudendal nerve. Although normal PNTML does not exclude partial damage, when prolonged, pudendal latencies seem to be reliably related to neuropathy.

Abnormally prolonged PNTML is usually found in patients with other pelvic floor disorders such as constipation with chronic straining, rectal prolapse, solitary rectal ulcer, and descending perineal syndrome. Neuropathy due to stretching of the pudendal nerve has been implicated, in theory, to explain the prolonged PNTML in those patients with chronic straining at stool. This entrapment/stretch theory is also thought to be the mechanism of pudendal lesion during vaginal delivery. However, a lack of correlation between perineal descent measurements and PNTML values has been demonstrated recently, and therefore other mechanisms may be involved.[25]

Anal endosonography

Anal endosonography has been proven useful for mapping IAS and EAS defects, and a high correlation with EMG mapping has been demonstrated in patients with traumatic fecal incontinence.[26] The different echogenic patterns of the anal sphincters facilitate their visualization during endosonography.

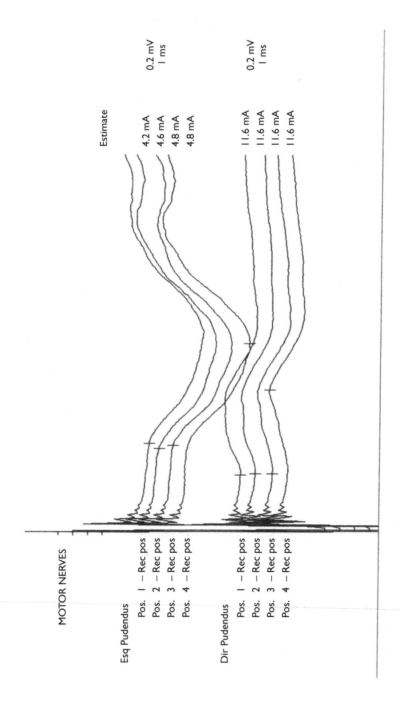

Figure 11.6 Abnormal pudendal nerve terminal motor latency (PNTML) on the left side (upper tracing).

The IAS is a 2–3 mm thick circular band and shows a uniform hypo-echogenicity. The puborectalis and the EAS, despite their mixed linear echogenicity, are both predominantly hyperechogenic, and the distinction is made by position, shape, and topography (Figure 11.7). Although unable to assess denervation, anal endosonography (by locating EAS and IAS defects) is better accepted by patients than EMG mapping (Figure 11.8). In addition, anal endosonography may be useful in detecting small perianal abscesses in patients with idiopathic anal pain and enteroceles.

Clinical application

Colonic transit study, anal manometry, cinedefecography, EMG, and PNTML assessment are considered standard physiologic studies. Through this physiologic investigation, treatable conditions of the colon, rectum, and anus can be diagnosed in 67% and 55% of patients with constipation and fecal incontinence, respectively.[1,2] In patients with rectal pain, however, these tests permit definite diagnosis in only 18%, and this condition remains poorly understood and refractory to therapy. In addition, these tests can be helpful preoperatively, whenever the anal continence status may be endangered due to the nature of the procedure or a pre-existent disorder affecting the mechanism of continence. In summary, physiologic testing permits objective assessment and post-therapeutic documentation of subjective functional colorectal disorders. Increasing experience with these methods will ensure a new perspective of evaluation of these highly prevalent and, at times, incapacitating symptoms. Finally, because the pelvic floor is an integrated functional structure, these disorders should be handled by a multidisciplinary approach, based on the intercommunication among urologists, gynecologists, gastroenterologists, neurologists, and colorectal surgeons.

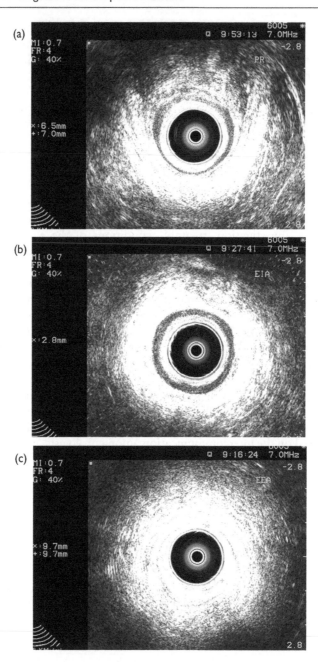

Figures 11.7 Normal echogenic patterns of the anal sphincters. (a) Puborectalis: U-shaped hyperechogenic band at the upper anal canal. (b) Internal anal sphincter: 2–3 mm thick hypoechogenic circular band. (c) External anal sphincter hyperechogenic circular band at the distal part of the anal canal.

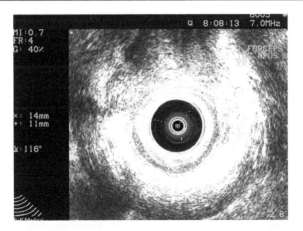

Figure 11.8 Anterior defect affecting both internal and external anal sphincters.

References

1. Wexner SD, Jorge JMN. Colorectal physiological tests: use or abuse of technology? Eur J Surg 1994;160:167–74.
2. Jorge JMN, Wexner SD. Physiologic evaluation. In: Wexner SD, Vernava AM, eds. Clinical decision making in colorectal surgery. New York: Igaku Shoin, 1995: 11–22.
3. Jorge JMN, Habr-Gama A. The value of sphincteric asymmetry index analysis in anal incontinence. Int J Colorectal Dis 2000;15:303–10.
4. Lestar B, Penninckx F, Kerremans R. The composition of anal basal pressure. An in vivo and in vitro study in man. Int J Colorect Dis 1989;4:118–22.
5. Marcello PW, Barrett RC, Coller JÁ, et al. Fatigue rate index as a new measurement of external sphincter function. Dis Colon Rectum 1998;41:336–43.
6. Habr-Gama A, Raia A, Correa Neto A. Motility of the sigmoid colon and rectum. Contribution to the physiopathology of megacolon in Chagas disease. Dis Colon Rectum 1971;14:291–304.
7. Metcalf AM, Phillips SF, Zinsmeister AR, et al. Simplified assessment of segmental colonic transit time. Gastroenterology 1987;92:40–7.
8. Hinton JM, Lennard-Jones JE, Young AC. A new method for studying gut transit times using radiopaque markers. Gut 1969;10:842–7.
9. Arhan P, Devroede G, Jehannin B, et al. Segmental colonic transit time. Dis Colon Rectum 1981;24:625–9.
10. Krishnamurthy S, Schuffler MD, Rohrmann CA, Pope CE II. Severe idiopathic constipation is associated with a distinctive abnormality of the colonic myenteric plexus. Gastroenterology 1985;88:26–34.
11. Wexner SD, Daniel N, Jagelman DG. Colectomy for constipation: physiologic investigation is the key to success. Dis Colon Rectum 1991;34:851–6.
12. Nam Y-S, Pikarsky AJ, Wexner SD, et al. Reproducibility of colonic transit study in patients with chronic constipation. Dis Colon Rectum 2001;44:86–92.

13. Finlay IG, Bartolo DCC, Bartram CI, et al. Symposium: Proctography. Int J Colorectal Dis 1988;3:67–89.
14. Karaus M, Neuhaus P, Wiedenmann B. Diagnosis of enteroceles by dynamic anorectal endosonography. Dis Colon Rectum 2000;43:1683–8.
15. Matsuoka H, Wexner SD, Desai MB, et al. A comparison between dynamic pelvic resonance imaging and videoproctography in patients with constipation. Dis Colon Rectum 2001;44:571–6.
16. Bartram CI, Turnbull GK, Lennard-Jones JE. Evaluation proctography: an investigation of rectal expulsion in 20 subjects without defecatory disturbance. Gastrointest Radiol 1988;13:72–80.
17. Wexner SD, Cheape JD, Jorge JMN, Heymen S, Jagelman DG. Prospective assessment of biofeedback for the treatment of paradoxical puborectalis syndrome. Dis Colon Rectum 1992;35:145–50.
18. Jorge JMN, Wexner SD, Ger GC, Jagelman DG. Cinedefecography and EMG in the diagnosis of nonrelaxing puborectalis syndrome. Dis Colon Rectum 1993;36:668–76.
19. Van Dam JH, Ginai AZ, Gosselink MJ, et al. Role of defecography in predicting clinical outcome of rectocele repair. Dis Colon Rectum 1997;40:201–7.
20. Johansson C, Nilsson BY, Holmstrom B, Dolk A, Mellgren A. Association between rectocele and paradoxical sphincter response. Dis Colon Rectum 1992;35:503–9.
21. Hawksworth W, Roux JP. Vaginal hysterectomy. J Obstet Gynecol 1958;63:214–28.
22. Jorge JM, Yang Y-K, Wexner SD. Incidence and clinical significance of sigmoidoceles as determined by a new classification system. Dis Colon Rectum 1994;37:1112–17.
23. Wexner SD, Marchetti F, Salanga VD, Corredor C, Jagelman DG. Neurophysiologic assessment of the anal sphincters. Dis Colon Rectum 1991;34:606–12.
24. Laurberg S, Swash M, Henry MM. Delayed external sphincter repair for obstetric tear. Br J Surg 1988;75:786–8.
25. Jorge JM, Wexner SD, Ehrenpreis ED, Nogueras JJ, Jagelman DG. Does perineal descent correlate with pudendal neuropathy? Dis Colon Rectum 1993;36:475–83.
26. Burnett SJ, Speakman CT, Kamm MA, Bartram CI. Confirmation of endosonographic detection of external anal sphincter defects by simultaneous electromyographic mapping. Br J Surg 1991;78:448–50.

Chapter 12

Management of urinary incontinence

Dharmesh S Kapoor and Gamal Ghoniem

Introduction

The commonest types of urinary incontinence presenting to the urologist and gynecologist are stress urinary incontinence (SUI) and that associated with detrusor overactivity (Figure 12.1). It is essential to differentiate between the two. This can be done by multichannel cystometry studies (CMG) or videofluorourodynamics (VFUD) (Figure 12.2).

Prevention

Control of obesity and pelvic floor exercises in the antenatal and post-partum period have been shown to reduce the risks of developing urinary incontinence.[1] Glazener et al[2] evaluated a randomly selected group of women at 3 months postpartum and found the incidence of UI to be 57% (>1/week). This had reduced by half at 12 months in women who had regular instructions in pelvic floor exercises.

Conservative treatment

Bladder diary

After assessing primary urine loss symptoms, an assessment of severity of incontinence is made by a 3- or 7-day bladder diary. The patient is asked to record oral liquid intake and timing of all the voids during the day. Episodes of urgency and incontinence are also recorded. This instrument provides baseline information and serves as a tool to monitor progress made during therapy. If urine loss-precipitating events are noted, additional useful information is obtained.

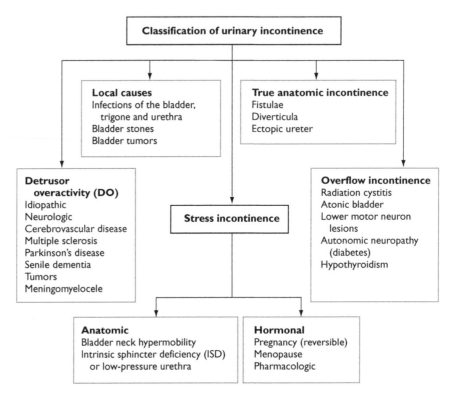

Figure 12.1 Classification of urinary incontinence.

Non-surgical Therapy

Bladder training

Bladder training is mainly used for women with overactive bladder (OAB). The main components of bladder training (or retraining) are patient education and timed voiding. The overall goals are increasing the interval between voids, with a concomitant reduction in the number of incontinent episodes. A target is set for a voiding interval of 1 hour in the first week, even if the woman has no desire to void. Pelvic floor contractions may be used to suppress sensations of urgency. Voiding intervals are increased incrementally by 15–30 minutes every week until the desired voiding interval of 2.5–3 hours is achieved. Bladder training has been found to be more effective than drug therapy or placebo as a first-line treatment of urgency-related incontinence.[3]

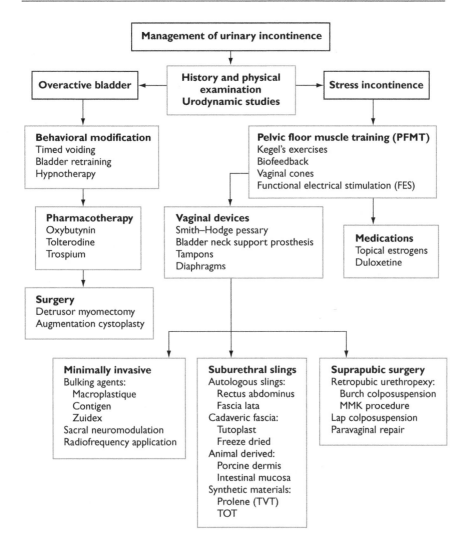

Figure 12.2 Management of urinary incontinence.

Pelvic floor muscle training

Pelvic floor muscle training (PFMT) is a well-established therapy in the management of urinary incontinence.[4] It is a widespread recommendation that PFMT should be offered as first-line conservative management to women with stress and/or mixed incontinence.

PFMT aims to isolate the levator muscles and contract them so as to be able to stop urination. A clinician should teach the patient to contract her pelvic floor muscles during a pelvic examination. The contractions are held for 10 seconds and are repeated at 15-second intervals. 'Quick flick' contractions are important for women with stress incontinence. The abdominal, buttock, and thigh muscles should be kept relaxed at all times. A patient may monitor her own progress by placing her index finger intravaginally while contracting her pelvic floor. Alternatively, a pneumatic perineometer maybe used to demonstrate strength of a pelvic floor contraction. Two-thirds of women whose initial treatment was successful and who were compliant in performing regular PFMT had favorable outcomes in a 10-year follow-up.[5]

Vaginal cones

Weighted vaginal cones are an aid to help women identify and train their pelvic floor muscles. These cones are tampon-sized and available in sets of five (or more) incremental weights. The lightest cone is initially inserted in the vagina, and the pelvic floor contracted during ambulation. Once the woman is able to retain a cone successfully, while ambulant, she proceeds to the next heavier cone. In a systematic review, cones were found to be as effective as PFMT, although adding the two modalities did not confer any benefit.[6] Discontinuation rates, however, are higher in women using cones.

Biofeedback

Biofeedback is defined as a behavioral treatment modality for incontinence used to teach acquisition of voluntary inhibition of detrusor contractions. Biofeedback is meant to promote greater selective control over pelvic floor muscles and reduce both stress and urge incontinence. Biofeedback techniques use vaginal or rectal pressure sensors or electromyography (EMG) electrodes. The patient is able to visualize actual pressure increases or EMG activity generated by each pelvic floor contraction. Simultaneous abdominal wall EMG helps patients identify Valsalva maneuvers that are counterproductive and may worsen incontinence. Data from one trial[7] suggest that women with biofeedback-assisted PFMT might experience more rapid improvement than PFMT alone. A subgroup that may benefit from biofeedback-assisted PFMT comprise those women who are not able to voluntarily contract their pelvic floor muscles at pretreatment assessment.[8] A randomized trial comparing biofeedback-assisted behavioral treatment with oxybutynin for urge incontinence found significantly more relief in the number of incontinence episodes and long-term continuity of treatment in the former group.[9]

Functional electrical stimulation

The proposed mechanism of functional electrical stimulation (FES) is alteration of lower urinary tract function by stimulation of the sacral autonomic or somatic nerves. There may also be a direct stimulatory effect on pelvic floor muscles and sphincters. The stimulation probe is placed in the vagina at the level of the pelvic musculature in the mid-vagina. During stimulation, the probe is held by the patient to prevent any migration and possible discomfort. FES current is pulsed: i.e. short periods of stimulation are alternated with rest periods. The strength of the stimulus is adjusted to avoid pain. Low frequency (10–20 Hz) is used for overactive bladder, mid-frequency (50–100 Hz) for stress incontinence, and high frequency (200 Hz) for urinary retention. A review of trials of FES for SUI showed cure in 18% and improvement in 34% of patients.[4] In the treatment of OAB, maximal electrostimulation cured 20% and improved 37% of women with urodynamic detrusor overactivity incontinence.[3] PFMT appears to offer greater benefit for women with genuine stress incontinence when compared with electrical stimulation. It might be that a particular subgroup of women with stress incontinence benefit from electrical stimulation, such as those who are unable to voluntarily contract the pelvic floor muscles. Similarly for OAB, electrostimulation is most beneficial to women who discontinue drugs due to side-effects.

Hypnotherapy

Freeman and Baxby first reported on the role of hypnotherapy for detrusor overactivity (DO).[10] They found a 96% cure or significant improvement rate at conclusion of treatment. When evaluated at 12 months, 70% of women continued to have symptom relief. They also demonstrated improvement in objective cystometric parameters in these women.

Medications

Overactive bladder medications

Overactive bladder is a debilitating condition that affects between 13% and 40% of the female population. Antimuscarinic drugs are currently the mainstay of treatment.

Oxybutynin is a musculotropic agent that acts distal to the cholinergic receptor. It acts as a smooth muscle relaxant, anticholinergic, and local anesthetic. Oxybutynin can be administered by various routes. Orally, a newer osmotic drug-delivery system is available that provides rate-controlled drug delivery over a 24-hour period. The decreased variation in peak-and-trough drug levels results in lesser side-effects. A 48% response rate is seen with oxybutynin when given as a rectal suppository. In those patients who self-catheterize and find the oral route intolerable, an intra-vesical route is also available. Since most side-effects are metabolite-related, a transdermal preparation is available that avoids first-pass metabolism in the liver and is claimed to reduce the incidence of dry mouth by 25%.

Tolterodine is another commonly used agent for treatment of OAB. It has a high selectivity for the urinary bladder, and is shown to have lesser side-effects. An extended-release preparation is available, which when used at night further decreases the side effects. Trospium chloride is a drug that is used as a second-line treatment for OAB. Newer drugs are now available including darifenacin (specific M_3 receptor blocker) and solifenacin. Although the newer drugs showed less side effects, their efficacy is slightly better.

Stress urinary incontinence medications

Duloxetine is a combined norepinephrine and serotonin reuptake inhibitor. It has recently been introduced as a treatment for stress and mixed urinary incontinence. Norepinephrine and serotonin stimulation of Onuf's nucleus receptors increases the activity in the pudendal nerve and produce urethral sphincter contraction mediated by acetylcholine. Recent studies have shown it to be superior to placebo.[11]

Non-surgical multimodality approaches

Combining various conservative modalities could result in synergistic beneficial effects. Indeed, when physical therapy modalities are combined with pharmacologic regimens, a 90% reduction in leakages has been noted in patients with detrusor overactivity.[12] In patients with stress urinary incontinence, duloxetine combined with PFMT showed a higher response than placebo, PFMT alone or duloxetine alone.[13]

Surgical therapy

A-detrusor hyperactivity

Sacral nerve neuromodulation (Interstim™)

Sacral nerve neuromodulation (InterStim) works by direct stimulation of the nerve roots in the sacral S3 foramen via an implanted electrode. A contraction of the external anal sphincter (anal wink) is observed when the S3 nerve root is stimulated. This contraction has latency 10 times longer than would be expected with a direct efferent stimulation, which shows that it is an afferent-mediated response. Sacral nerve stimulation has been shown to be effective in the treatment of urge urinary incontinence.[14]

Surgical options for intractable destrusor overactivity

Surgical options for DO include detrusor myomectomy and augmentation cystoplasty: the latter is more successful, with published success rates between

70% and 90%.[15] However, there are significant morbidities associated with surgery, and not all women are willing to opt for this alternative (Table 12.1). Neuromodulation is a promising minimally invasive therapy for such patients.

B-stress urinary incontinence

Colposuspension

Burch colposuspension remains one of the most effective surgical procedures for stress incontinence with continence achieved in 85–90% at 1 year and 70% at 5 years. The common side-effects are voiding difficulties in 10%, de-novo detrusor overactivity in 17%, and enterocele and rectocele formation in 14%.[16] A concomitant cystocele can also be treated by a colposuspension. Laparoscopic colposuspension has been shown to have similar results in the medium term. However, there are no long-term data on its efficacy.

Paravaginal repair

This procedure is based on the suburethral 'hammock' support hypothesis. It presumes that breaks in the attachment of the endopelvic fascia to the arcus tendineus fascia pelvis (ATFP) cause stress incontinence. Paravaginal repair consists of reattachment of the fascia to the ATFP. Whereas a cohort study reported a 97% success rate, the only randomized study showed it to be inferior to colposuspension (100% vs 72%).[17]

Anterior vaginal repair

Anterior repair (with Kelly bladder buttress sutures) has disappointing long-term results in the treatment of stress incontinence, and is not recommended. It still has a role in the treatment of prolapse.

Table 12.1 Complications of surgical treatment for stress incontinence

Complication	Colposuspension	Pubovaginal slings	TVT	TOT[a]
Bladder/urethral injury	0–3%	0–10%	5%	0–2%
De-novo OAB	10–20%	2–20%	4–15%	12%
Voiding problems	5–20%	10	5–25%	14%
Tape erosion	NA	5–16%	0–2%	0
Vascular injury	3%	?	0–2%	N/L
Prolapse	3–29%	NA	NA	NA

TVT = tension-free vaginal taping, TOT = transobturator taping, OAB = overactive bladder.
[a] Only one prospective randomized trial.

Needle suspension

Modifications of Pereyra's original technique (including Stamey, Raz, bone anchor systems) have a lower continence rate and a higher complication rate. This technique has largely been superseded by sling operations.

Sling procedures

The suburethral (or pubovaginal) slings are highly effective options for primary treatment and for previously failed surgery. Materials used include autologous (rectus sheath, fascia lata), allografts (cadaveric fascia lata), xenografts (porcine dermal implants, porcine intestinal mucosa), and synthetic materials like prolene. Complications include vaginal erosion (16%), urethral erosion (0–5%), and voiding difficulty (2%).

Tension-free vaginal taping

Tension-free vaginal taping (TVT; Gynecare, Ethicon Inc., Somerville, NJ) is one of the most popular methods of surgically restoring urinary continence. It involves placement of a Prolene tape around the mid-urethra via a minimal vertical anterior vaginal incision. The tape is brought out through two suprapubic incisions. Check cystoscopy is performed after tape insertion to detect bladder or urethral perforations. Should a perforation occur, the tape is withdrawn and reinserted. Once perforations have been excluded, the vaginal and the suprapubic incisions are closed with absorbable sutures. TVT can be performed under local anesthetic as well as regional and general anesthesia. The procedure results in minimal blood loss, and can be done in a day-care setting. Major complications are rare and include bowel and vascular injury. TVT is often combined with prolapse repair surgery. In these cases, it is prudent to leave a suprapubic or urethral catheter in situ. Voiding trial is commenced shortly afterwards and the catheter removed once the post-void residual is less than 100 ml. In a recent randomized trial, TVT has been shown to have higher cure rates than colposuspension at 2-year follow-up.[18]

Transobturator taping

Transobturator taping (TOT) is a relatively newer technique for management of urinary incontinence. Since the tape is brought out through the obturator foramen into the thigh, it is believed to eliminate the risks of bowel and vascular injury associated with the TVT. A small randomized trial with 1-year follow-up found TOT to be as effective as the TVT, with no major complications reported.[19]

Bulking agents

Bulking agents are usually injected via a cystoscope into the bladder neck. Bulking agents such as Contigen (Bard Inc., Covington, GA) and Durasphere (Carbon Medical Technologies, St Paul, MN) have been used in the treatment of incontinence for both the urethral and anal sphincters. They are believed to work by increasing the resting pressure and tone of the sphincters. The success rates of both these agents in the treatment of urinary incontinence was 63% at 1 year and 33% at 4 years, respectively.[20]

Macroplastique (Uroplasty BV, Netherlands) has reported success rates of 60% in women with recurrent SUI.[21]

Radiofrequency bladder neck suspension

Radiofrequency application is a new treatment for genuine stress urinary incontinence. The purported mechanism is a thermal effect on the collagenated tissue within the endopelvic fascia at the bladder neck. This causes shrinkage of the fascia, thereby reducing bladder neck hypermobility. Radiofrequency has been used in trials both vaginally and laparoscopically with cure/improvement rates of 73–83% at 1 year.[22,23] However, long-term data are needed on safety and efficacy before it can be commended to clinical practice.

Artificial sphincters

Artificial sphincters are mainly used after failed continence surgery. Although the success rate for this indication is high (92%), there is high morbidity and need for revision surgery (17%) due to cuff erosion or device malfunction.[24]

References

1. Baessler K, Schuessler B. Childbirth-induced trauma to the urethral continence mechanism: review and recommendations. Urology 2003;62:39–44.
2. Glazener CMA, Herbison GP, Wilson PD, et al. Conservative management of persistent postnatal urinary and faecal incontinence: randomised controlled trial. BMJ 2001;323:1–5.
3. Berghmans LC, Hendriks HJ, DeBie RA, et al. Conservative treatment of urge urinary incontinence in women: a systematic review of randomised clinical trials. BJU Int 2000;85:254–63.
4. Berghmans LC, Hendriks HJ, Bo K, et al. Conservative treatment of stress urinary incontinence in women: a systematic review of randomised clinical trials. Br J Urol 1998;82:181–91.
5. Cammu H, Van Nylen M, Amy JJ. A 10-year follow-up after Kegel pelvic floor muscle exercises for genuine stress incontinence. BJU Int 2000;85:655–8.
6. Herbison P, Plevnik S, Mantle J. Weighted vaginal cones for urinary incontinence. Cochrane Database Syst Rev 2000;CD002114.

7. Berghmans LC, Frederiks CM, de Bie RA, et al. Efficacy of biofeedback, when included with pelvic floor muscle exercise treatment, for genuine stress incontinence. Neurourol Urodyn 1996;15:37–52.

8. Burns PA, Pranikoff K, Nochajski T, Desotelle P, Harwood MK. Treatment of stress incontinence with pelvic floor exercises and biofeedback. J Am Geriatr Soc 1990;38:341–4.

9. Burgio KL, Locher JL, Goode PS, et al. Behavioral vs drug treatment for urge urinary incontinence in older women: a randomised controlled trial. JAMA 1998;280:1995–2000.

10. Freeman RM, Baxby K. Hypnotherapy for incontinence caused by the unstable detrusor. Br Med J 1982;284:1831–4.

11. Dmochowski RR. Duloxetine versus placebo for treatment of North American women with stress urinary incontinence. J Urol 2003;170:1259–63.

12. Davila GW, Bernier F. Multimodality pelvic physiotherapy treatment of urinary incontinence in adult women. Int Urogynecol J 1995;6:187–94.

13. Ghoniem GM, Leeuwen JSV, Elser DM et al. A radomized controlled trial of duloxetine alone, pelvic floor muscle training alone, combined treatment and no active treatment in women with stress urinary incontinence. J Urol 2005; 173:1647–53.

14. Bosch JL, Groen J. Sacral (S3) segmental nerve stimulation as a treatment for urge-incontinence in patients with detrusor instability: results of chronic electrical stimulation using an implantable neuroprosthesis. J Urol 1995; 154:504–7.

15. Flood HD, Malhotra SJ, O'Connell HE, et al. Long-term results and complications using augmentation cystoplasty in reconstructive urology. Neurourol Urodyn 1995;14:297–309.

16. Colombo M, Zanetta G, Vitobello D, Milani R. The Burch colposuspension for women with detrusor overactivity. Br J Obstet Gynaecol 1996;103:255–60.

17. Lapitan MC, Cody DJ, Grant AM. Open retropubic colposuspension for urinary incontinence in women. Cochrane Database Syst Rev 2003;CD002912.

18. Ward KL, Hilton P. A prospective multicenter randomized trial of tension-free vaginal tape and colposuspension for primary urodynamic stress incontinence: two year follow-up. Am J Obstet Gynecol 2004;190:324–31.

19. deTayrac R, Deffieux X, Droupy S, et al. A prospective randomized trial comparing tension-free vaginal tape and transobturator suburethral tape for surgical treatment of stress urinary incontinence. Am J Obstet Gynecol 2004;190:602–8.

20. Chrouser KL, Fick F, Goel A, et al. Carbon coated zirconium beads in beta-glucan gel and bovine glutaraldehyde cross-linked collagen injections for intrinsic sphincter deficiency: continence and satisfaction after extended follow-up. J Urol 2004;171:1152–5.

21. Radley SC, Chapple CR, Mitsogiannis IC, Glass KS. Transurethral implantation of macroplastique for the treatment of female stress urinary incontinence secondary to urethral sphincter deficiency. Eur Urol 2001;39:383–9.

22. Dmochowski RR, Avon M, Ross J, et al. Transvaginal radio frequency treatment of the endopelvic fascia: a prospective evaluation for the treatment of genuine stress urinary incontinence. J Urol 2003;169:1028–32.

23. Fulmer BR, Sakamoto K, Turk TM, et al. Acute and long-term outcomes of radio frequency bladder neck suspension. J Urol 2002;16:141–5.

24. Webster SD, Perez LM, Khoury JM, Timmons SL. Management of type 3 stress urinary incontinence using artificial urinary sphincter. Urology 1992; 39:499–503.

Chapter 13

Management of genital prolapse

Daniel Biller and G Willy Davila

Introduction

The incidence of genital prolapse is estimated to be 25% when the leading edge of the prolapse is at the hymen or below.[1] Management is determined by multiple factors, including concomitant compartmental defects, co-incidence of incontinence, and patient goals and expectations. Conservative therapy consists of space-occupying pessaries. Surgical therapy incorporates principles of abdominal wall hernia repair applied to advanced vaginal and pelvic reconstructive procedures.

Surgical correction of vaginal prolapse can be accomplished through a vaginal, abdominal, or laparoscopic approach. The appropriate surgical approach is determined by several factors, including the preoperative evaluation of concomitant vaginal support defects, the presence of incontinence, history of previous pelvic surgery, the patient's surgical risk, and the surgeon's training and skill level.

Non-surgical therapy

Pessary

The increase in the elderly population requiring conservative treatment of prolapse has led to a resurgence of pessary use. Pessaries function as intravaginal space-occupying devices, which hold the pelvic organs in place. Multiple different shapes and sizes are available, and have indications for treatment of prolapse as well as stress urinary incontinence. Clinical use of the pessary is based on a 'best fit, trial and error' process. The best pessary elevates the prolapse and remains in place during ambulation. It should rest comfortably in the vaginal canal without causing pain or obstructing voiding or bowel function. For advanced prolapse, Gelhorn pessaries work best, although ring pessaries may be easier to insert and remove.

Pessary care recommendations should be followed closely for safe long-term use. For patients able to remove and reinsert the pessary, the device may be removed nightly or at least two nights per week. Follow-up with the clinician should be every 6 months to assure vaginal mucosal health and proper fit and placement. The patient who is unable to care for the pessary herself must be seen by the clinician on a regular basis every 6–8 weeks for pessary cleaning and reinsertion and vaginal mucosal examination. Patients must be encouraged to use intravaginal estrogen regularly to prevent vaginal ulceration from foreign body use within the vagina, especially the postmenopausal patient. The typical dosage is 1 g inserted with an applicator two nights per week. This low dosage does not result in systemic absorption of estradiol.[2]

Surgical therapy

Repair of the anterior wall (cystocele)

The successful management of anterior vaginal wall prolapse remains one of the greatest challenges for the pelvic reconstructive surgeon. The anterior vaginal wall is the compartment most likely to demonstrate recurrent prolapse after reconstructive surgery, with recurrence rates as high as 20%.[3,4]

Advanced anterior vaginal prolapse can result from defects in several areas of pelvic support including:

1. attenuation or tears of the vaginal fibromuscular layer (fascia) in the midline (central defect)
2. loss of lateral attachments from the anterior vagina to the pelvic sidewall (lateral or paravaginal defect)
3. loss of bladder neck support
4. separation of the fibromuscular layer (fascia) transversely from the vaginal apex.

Recent observations have shown that this last anatomic alteration probably occurs with the greatest frequency. More importantly, lack of reattachment of this layer to the vaginal apex is probably responsible for most cystocele recurrences postoperatively.

Anterior colporrhaphy

Anterior vaginal prolapse resulting from a central defect is best corrected through a transvaginal approach. The anterior colporrhaphy was popularized by Howard Kelly in 1912, and although no longer an acceptable treatment for stress urinary incontinence, it still remains a commonly used technique for transvaginal correction of anterior vaginal prolapse. A midline vaginal incision is made, and dissection is carried laterally to separate the vaginal epithelium from the endopelvic fascia to each lateral sulcus.

After completing the dissection, the endopelvic fascia is plicated in the midline, thereby repairing the central defect and elevating the bladder base and anterior vagina. The bladder neck can be preferentially supported by further plicating the periurethral tissue underneath the bladder neck (Kelly plication). Most importantly, the plicated fascia *must* be reattached to the vaginal apex. The excess vaginal epithelium is then trimmed and the incision is closed. A 2-0 polyglycolic acid Vicryl suture is used. A vaginal pack is then placed for postoperative hemostasis.

Outcomes of the traditional anterior colporrhaphy are largely limited to retrospective reviews and case series. The reported recurrence rates after anterior vaginal wall prolapse repair have been high (range: 0 to 59%).[3–5]

Paravaginal defect repair

The goal of the paravaginal defect repair is to correct anterior vaginal wall prolapse that results from loss of lateral support by reattaching the lateral vaginal sulcus to its normal lateral attachment site (arcus tendineus fascia pelvis (ATFP) or white line of the pelvic sidewall). Paravaginal defect repairs can be performed retropubically or vaginally.

Abdominal approach

The retropubic space is entered through an abdominal incision, and the bladder is retracted medially to expose the paravaginal space. The obturator fossa, neurovascular bundle, and ischial spine are identified. The surgeon's nondominant hand is then placed into the vagina and used to elevate the lateral superior vaginal sulcus to its site of normal attachment along the course of the ATFP. Four to six simple interrupted stitches of nonabsorbable suture (No. 0 polypropylene) are used to reattach the lateral vagina to the ATFP bilaterally. The first suture is placed through full thickness (excluding the vaginal epithelium) of the lateral vaginal apex and then through the ATFP just anterior to the ischial spine. Additional sutures are placed at 1 cm intervals through the lateral vaginal wall and along the entire course of the ATFP to the inferior edge of the pubic symphysis.

Vaginal approach

Transvaginal paravaginal repair can be more challenging than the abdominal approach; however, it avoids an abdominal incision and facilitates concurrent central defect repair for those patients with midline and lateral support defects.

A midline vertical incision is made through the vaginal epithelium from the mid-urethra to the vaginal apex. The vaginal epithelium is then sharply dissected off the underlying endopelvic fascia, and the dissection is continued laterally to the pelvic sidewall and to the level of the ischial spine.

Visualization of the adipose tissue of the retropubic space confirms the presence of a paravaginal defect; the normal lateral attachment of the anterior vaginal wall would preclude this. Four to six interrupted nonabsorbable sutures (No. 0 polypropylene) are placed through the ATFP and lateral vaginal wall sulcus from the level of the ischial spine to the pubic symphysis at 1 cm intervals and then sequentially tied.

The success rate of paravaginal defect repair for treatment of anterior vaginal prolapse is limited to case series and retrospective reviews. Limited reports of abdominal paravaginal repair demonstrate anatomic success rates ranging from 92% to 97%.[6] Reports of vaginal paravaginal repair demonstrate success rates of 76–100%.[7] There are few long-term data on laparoscopic paravaginal repair for the treatment of anterior vaginal prolapse.

Studies that have differentiated lateral from central recurrence have revealed that a central recurrence (22–25%) is more common than a lateral recurrence (2–8%).[8] To date, there are no studies comparing paravaginal defect repair with or without midline anterior repair to traditional anterior colporrhaphy alone.

Rectocele

Rectoceles arise from a tear or stretching of the rectovaginal fascia, resulting in defects in the integrity of the rectovaginal septum, and herniation of the rectal wall into the vaginal lumen. Although there are high rates of anatomic cures, there are conflicting reports with regard to functional outcome, and many report postoperative dyspareunia. Gynecologic surgeons perform this operation on a frequent basis by itself or in conjunction with other pelvic reconstructive procedures. The restoration of normal anatomy to the lower posterior vaginal wall is referred to as a posterior repair or colporrhaphy.

Although frequently used interchangeably with the term rectocele repair, the two operations may have vastly different treatment goals. Whereas a rectocele repair focuses on repairing herniation of the anterior rectal wall into the vaginal canal, which is due to a weakness in the rectovaginal septum, a posterior colporrhaphy is designed to correct a bulge, if it is present, as well as provide structural integrity to the posterior vaginal wall and introitus. A modified repair, the discrete fascial defect repair, shows promising anatomic and functional results.

Posterior colporrhaphy technique

Posterior colporrhaphy is commonly performed in conjunction with a perineoplasty to address a relaxed perineum and widened genital hiatus. Allis clamps are placed on the hymen bilaterally and then approximated in the midline. The resultant vagina should loosely admit two to three fingers. A triangular skin incision is made between the Allis clamps, and sharp dissection is then performed to separate the posterior vaginal mucosa from the underlying rectovaginal fascia. A midline incision is made along the length of the vagina to a site above the superior edge of the rectocele. The dissection is carried laterally to the lateral vaginal sulcus and medial margins of the puborectalis muscles. The rectovaginal fascia with or without the underlying levator ani muscles is then plicated with interrupted sutures while depressing the anterior rectal wall. A concomitant perineoplasty may be performed by plicating the bulbocavernosus and transverse perineii muscles. This reinforces the perineal body and provides enhanced support to the corrected rectocele.

Discrete fascial defect repair technique

The intent of the discrete fascial defect repair of rectoceles is to identify all present fascial tears and reapproximate their edges. The surgical dissection is similar to the traditional posterior colporrhaphy, whereby the vaginal mucosa is dissected off the underlying rectovaginal fascia to the lateral border of the levator muscles. However, instead of plicating the fascia and levator muscles in the midline, the fascial tears are identified and repaired with interrupted permanent sutures. A perineoplasty may be necessary if an enlarged vaginal hiatus is present. Long-term results of site-specific rectocele repairs are not available.

Enterocele

Enterocele has been defined as a peritoneum-lined sac herniating through the vaginal wall, most commonly between the vagina and rectum. Women with an enterocele often have concomitant vaginal support defects. Symptoms are often complex and cannot be attributed solely to the enterocele. Nonetheless, women with large enteroceles often complain of pelvic pressure, fullness, vaginal protrusion, and low backache.

Surgical repair of enterocele can be performed vaginally, abdominally, or laparoscopically, but few data exist comparing the various repair techniques. Surgical approach and procedure depend on the presence of concomitant pathology and the surgeon's skill and preference.

Traditional vaginal enterocele repair includes isolation of the entero-cele sac, careful exploration of its contents, and closure with multiple circumferential, nonabsorbable, purse-string sutures incorporating the cardinal–uterosacral ligaments.

Vaginal enterocele repair

Enterocele usually coexists with other support defects, and concurrent vagi-nal vault suspension, cystocele, and rectocele repair are often necessary. Access to the enterocele is gained in a similar fashion to the posterior col-porrhaphy by separating the endopelvic fascia from the posterior vaginal epithelium to the level just distal to the vaginal apex. The enterocele is iden-tified as a fascial separation from the vaginal apex. The defect can be cor-rected using several interrupted permanent sutures. When the enterocele sac is difficult to distinguish from the rectum, differentiation is aided by a rec-tal examination with simultaneous dissection of the enterocele sac from the rectal wall.

In a traditional enterocele repair, after the enterocele sac has been dis-sected from the vagina and rectum, traction is placed on it with two Allis clamps and the sac is entered sharply. The enterocele sac is explored digi-tally and any adhesions are dissected to the level of its neck. Under direct visualization, circumferential, nonabsorbable purse-string sutures are used to close the enterocele sac. The cardinal–uterosacral ligaments may be incorporated as well. The sutures are sequentially tied. Care should be taken to avoid kinking the ureters, and cystoscopy is recommended.

Modified McCall culdoplasty

McCall described the technique of surgical correction of enterocele and vault suspension at the time of vaginal hysterectomy. The McCall culdoplasty closes the redundant cul-de-sac and associated enterocele, provides apical support, and lengthens the vagina.

After hysterectomy a permanent suture (silk or Prolene) is used to suture together the uterosacral ligaments along with intervening peritoneum and full thickness of the vaginal epithelium posteriorly at the apex. The sutures should be placed through the uterosacral ligaments at a distance from the cuff equal to the amount of vaginal vault prolapse that is present (Figure 13.1). This will then resupport the vaginal apex to a satisfactory level. We use the general formula based on the POP-Q examination of TVL−D to determine how many centimeters above the cuff to place the sutures. In cases of advanced vault prolapse, two or three McCall sutures may be nec-essary. Success rates with McCall culdoplasties are quite high, and pelvic surgeons performing vaginal hysterectomies are encouraged to routinely

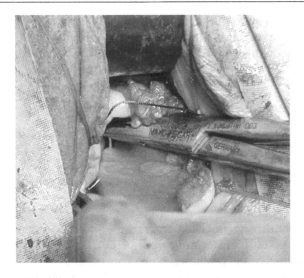

Figure 13.1 McCall culdoplasty at the time of vaginal hysterectomy. Sutures are placed along the uterosacral ligaments such that vaginal length (TVL) is normalized according to point C and D on the preoperative POP-Q examination.

perform McCall culdoplasties as part of a vaginal hysterectomy. Cystoscopy is recommended to assure ureteral patency.

Vaginal vault prolapse

Prolapse of the vaginal apex is considered to be an increasingly common anatomic alteration, and is present in most cases of advanced prolapse. It is likely that in the past, most cases of vaginal vault prolapse were not identified properly, resulting in prompt recurrence of prolapse following a traditional 'A&P repair.' In the post-hysterectomy patient, there is usually a band of scar tissue at the vaginal apex with two dimples on either side representing the previous attachments of the uterosacral or cardinal ligaments. Various options are available for surgical management of vaginal vault prolapse.

Uterosacral ligament suspension

Analogous to a McCall culdoplasty, identification of the uterosacral ligaments and reattachment of the ligaments to the vaginal cuff can result in a physiologic axis and is the preferred route of vault suspension for many surgeons. In cases of mild vault prolapse, this procedure can be readily performed as the uterosacral ligaments can be easily identified. However, in cases of more advanced vaginal vault prolapse, identifying the uterosacral ligaments can be quite difficult and there is an increased risk of ureteral injury. The rate of ureteral injury is reported to be between 11% and 13%.[9] The longevity of this technique has not been demonstrated in published series.

Ileococcygeus suspension

Elevation of the vaginal apex to the ileococcygeus muscle along the pelvic sidewall may represent the simplest way of addressing vault prolapse. Permanent, monofilament sutures are placed through the vaginal epithelium into the ileococcygeus muscle and its fascia and tied on either apical sidewall to resuspend the apex. The simplicity of this technique is attractive as a full dissection of the vaginal wall is not necessary. However, this technique will not correct associated anterior and posterior vaginal wall prolapse in most cases. Its main utility will be in the management of isolated unilateral vaginal vault prolapse, which can occur following a unilateral sacrospinous fixation, or from a unilateral high paravaginal detachment. In a patient who is not sexually active, the presence of a monofilament suture at the vaginal apex should not be associated with dyspareunia and should not cause significant granulation tissue. Therefore, this procedure is probably most useful as an adjunct procedure for a patient with an isolated apical unilateral defect.

Sacrospinous fixation

Elevation of the vaginal apex to the sacrospinous ligament is one of the most commonly performed vaginal approach vault suspension procedures. It can be performed unilaterally or bilaterally based on surgeon preference. The pararectal space is entered after a posterior wall dissection and the ischial spine and sacrospinous ligament extending from the spine to the sacrum is identified. The underside of the vaginal apex is then sutured to the sacrospinous ligament. Traditionally, it is performed on the right side. The bilateral approach may provide a more physiologic correction of vaginal vault prolapse (Figure 13.2). Any additional reconstructive procedures are then performed. It is important to place the sutures through rather than around the sacrospinous ligament, as the pudendal nerve, artery, and vein are located immediately deep to the sacrospinous ligament and significant morbidity can occur if those structures are damaged. There have been no other significant complications with this procedure, including no significant bowel dysfunction with the bilateral approach. The success rate of the sacrospinous fixation and restoration of vaginal vault support is over 90% in multiple series.[3] The main concern with this procedure is the fact that the vagina is placed in an exaggerated horizontal position. This nonphysiologic axis results in a higher rate of cystocele formation, reported at around

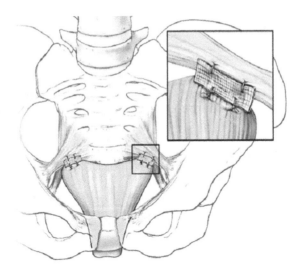

Figure 13.2 Sacrospinous fixation can be performed bilaterally, attaching the vaginal apices to the ipsilateral sacrospinous ligaments.

20–30%.[5,10] In addition, if an anti-incontinence procedure is performed along with a sacrospinous fixation, the rate of voiding dysfunction can be elevated due to the pulling of the vagina in an anterior-to-posterior direction by both repairs.

Posterior intravaginal slingplasty/vault suspension

A more recent approach for the restoration of vault support is the use of a synthetic mesh tape to recreate suspensory ligaments. This technique follows similar principles to those for urinary anti-incontinence minimally invasive mid-urethral tension-free slings. For the posterior intravaginal slingplasty (IVS), a posterior vaginal dissection is performed to the level of the vaginal apex. The tape to be secured to the vaginal apex is then placed through bilateral pararectal incisions approximately 3 cm lateral and 3 cm posterior to the anus. A metal tunneler is guided through the levator muscles and onto the endopelvic fascia over the ileococcygeus muscle or immediately anterior to the ischial spine and sacrospinous ligament (Figure 13.3). Once the tape has healed, it becomes a new suspensory ligament for the vaginal apex. This technique has been noted to result in a more physiologic vaginal axis and normal post-hysterectomy vaginal length.[11] Its newness precludes any objective long-term evaluation.

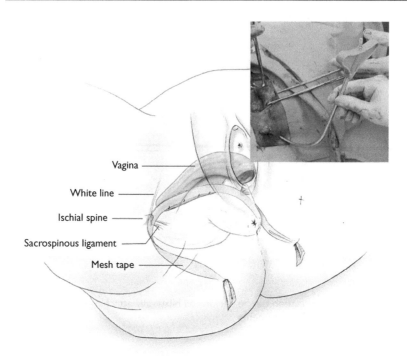

Vagina

White line

Ischial spine

Sacrospinous ligament

Mesh tape

Figure 13.3 Posterior intravaginal slingplasty (IVS). The vaginal apex is suspended to the tape placed from pelvic sidewall to pelvic sidewall using the Tunneler device.

Abdominal approaches to vaginal vault prolapse

Abdominal sacrocolpopexy

Suspension of the vaginal apex to the sacral promontory utilizing a graft bridge is considered by most surgeons to be the gold standard procedure for vaginal vault prolapse (Figure 13.4). Although it requires an abdominal incision, the resultant anatomy carries the highest longevity and least risk of sexual dysfunction and dyspareunia. The procedure entails performing an abdominal incision and exposing the sacral promontory by incising the peritoneum between the right ureter and the sigmoid colon. The periosteum is cleared of any connective tissue. Two or three (2-0 Prolene) sutures are then placed through the periosteum. Since significant life-threatening bleeding has been reported in this area, an option is to place bone anchors with an attached suture to secure the graft to the sacral promontory periosteum. This technique may minimize problematic bleeding. Once the sutures have been placed through the periosteum, the vaginal apex is identified with an EEA obturator or the operator's hand. The vault is identified and the peritoneum and bladder are dissected off the anterior vaginal wall. Along the posterior vaginal wall, any fascial defects are identified and the rectal reflection is clearly noted. The graft to be utilized for the vault suspension should be a synthetic polypropylene graft. It should have a long arm for the posterior wall and a shorter arm for the anterior vaginal wall. This can be fashioned from a standard piece of polypropylene mesh folded in half. Typically, three rows of 2-0 polypropylene sutures are placed along the back wall of the vagina and two rows along the front wall of the vagina. Once these are secured to the graft, the graft can then be suspended to the sacral promontory with minimal tension. Prior to suspending the graft, the posterior cul-de-sac should be obliterated either by a uterosacral ligament plication or a Halban/Moscowitz technique. If a biologic graft is utilized for this technique, the failure rate is significantly increased. Once the vault has been suspended, any additional necessary reconstructive procedures can be performed. These typically include a paravaginal repair as well as posterior colporrhaphy.

Sacrocolpopexy is associated with a greater risk of ileus formation. It is thus important to feed these patients very slowly.

Success of the sacrocolpopexy approach is 90–98% in multiple series. Besides ileus and bleeding complications, mesh erosion has been reported in

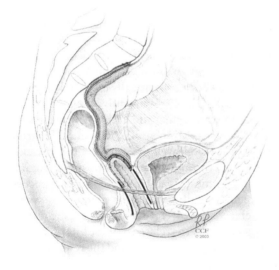

Figure 13.4 Abdominal sacrocolpopexy entails placement of a suspensory mesh bridge from the vaginal apex to the sacral promontory periosteum.

a small percentage of patients. If polypropylene mesh is utilized, this can be simply trimmed in the office or operating room and the epithelial defect closed.

Laparoscopic sacrocolpopexy

In the hands of a surgeon who is skilled in laparoscopic surgery and has an appropriately trained team, the procedure can be performed laparoscopically in an identical fashion to the open procedure. The long-term results of the laparoscopic procedure are not known at this time and the procedure can be technically difficult. However, recovery time may be reduced.

Laparoscopic uterosacral ligament suspension

A simpler laparoscopic approach to vault suspension involves plicating the uterosacral ligaments and the intervening vaginal apex with 1–3 rows of 2-0 polypropylene sutures. This can be achieved laparoscopically with extracorporeal knot-tying. This technique can be carried out by most surgeons who perform laparoscopic surgery. Success rates may be lower for a woman with significant intraperitoneal scarring or advanced degrees of prolapse. However, it is a very useful technique for women with mild to moderate uterine prolapse without cervical hypertrophy, as well as for women with mild to moderate vaginal vault prolapse. Care must be taken to identify the ureters during placement of the sutures.

Kits for vaginal prolapse surgery

Recent advances in reconstructive surgery include the development of kits to correct multiple defects simultaneously. The intent of these kits is to standardize surgical approaches utilizing specifically designed needles and permanent or biologic mesh grafts. Two kits are currently available, the Apogee (for vaginal apical and posterior wall repair) and Perigee (for anterior wall repair) kits (American Medical Systems, Minnetonka, MN) and the Prolift total vaginal mesh reconstruction kit (Gynecare Ethicon, New Brunswick, NJ). These kits are designed to be placed through anterior or posterior vaginal wall incisions and dissections and the mesh is anchored to the ileococcygeus muscle or sacrospinous ligament apically, obturator membrane anteriorly, and perineum. Multiple defects are corrected simultaneously, resulting in potential time savings in surgery. Concerns related to these kits involve the large amount of synthetic or biologic mesh that is used and the required surgeon training in order to be able to safely perform these procedures. Nevertheless, the future holds for standardization of surgical techniques for correction of vaginal prolapse by surgeons' utilization of pre-fabricated kits which are designed to correct all anatomical defects at one setting.

Grafts for prolapse surgery

Recently, the use of grafts has been popularized for the enhancement of the longevity of reconstructive procedures. Both synthetic (i.e. polypropylene, Vicryl) and biologic (i.e. cadaveric fascia lata or dermis, bovine pericardium, porcine dermis, small intestinal submucosa) grafts are available and are used for most reconstructive procedures. Safety and efficacy have not been determined, and thus routine use cannot be recommended.

Conclusions

Pelvic reconstructive surgery is evolving from surgery with a greater emphasis on art to an evolving science. Multiple techniques, which improve long-term success rates, are being developed. Proper preoperative evaluation and assessment of prolapse segments are crucial to performance of the correct surgical procedure for an individual patient.

References

1. Nygaard I, Bradley C, Brandt D. Women's Health Initiative. Pelvic organ prolapse in older women: prevalence and risk factors. Obstet Gynecol 2004;104(3):489–97.
2. Handa VL, Bachus KE, Johnston WW, Robboy SJ, Hammond CB. Vaginal administration of low-dose conjugated estrogens: systemic absorption and effects on the endometrium. Obstet Gynecol 1994;84(2):215–18.
3. Morley GW, DeLancey JOL. Sacrospinous ligament fixation for eversion of the vagina. Am J Obstet Gynecol 1988;158:872–81.
4. Shull BL, Benn SJ, Kuehl TJ. Surgical management of prolapse of the anterior vaginal segment: an analysis of support defects, operative morbidity, and anatomic outcome. Am J Obstet Gynecol 1994;171:1429–39
5. Shull BL, Capen CV, Riggs MW, Kuehl TJ. Preoperative and postoperative analysis of site-specific pelvic support defects in 81 women treated with sacrospinous ligament suspension and pelvic reconstruction. Am J Obstet Gynecol 1992;166:1764–71.
6. Shull BL, Baden WF. A six-year experience with paravaginal defect repair for stress urinary incontinence. Am J Obstet Gynecol. 1989;160:1432–40.
7. Young SB, Daman JJ, Bony LG. Vaginal paravaginal repair: one-year outcome. Am J Obstet Gynecol 2001;185(6):1360–6.
8. Elkins TE, Chesson RR, Videla F, et al. Transvaginal paravaginal repair: a useful adjunctive procedure in pelvic relaxation surgery. J Pelvic Surg 2000; 6:11–15.
9. Barber MD, Visco AG, Weidner AC, Amundsen CL, Bump RC. Bilateral uterosacral ligament vaginal vault suspension with site-specific endopelvic fascia defect repair for treatment of pelvic organ prolapse. Am J Obstet Gynecol 2000;183(6):1402–10; discussion 1410–1.

10. Paraiso MF, Ballard LA, Walters MD, Lee JC, Mitchinson AR. Pelvic support defects and visceral and sexual function in women treated with sacrospinous ligament suspension and pelvic reconstruction. Am J Obstet Gynecol 1996;175(6):1423–30; discussion 1430–1.
11. Davila GW, Miller D. Vaginal vault suspension using the posterior IVS technique. J Pelvic Med Surg 2004;10(1):539.

Chapter 14

Management of fecal incontinence and rectal prolapse

Oded Zmora, Hagit Tulchinsky, and Yishai Ron

Introduction

Although fecal incontinence and rectal prolapse may both result from attenuated pelvic floor and may coexist, the surgical approach to these conditions frequently differs, and thus in this chapter we will discuss these two
conditions separately.

Fecal incontinence

Very few benign conditions cause embarrassment and jeopardize the physical, mental, and social quality of life as much as the inability to control
bowel function. The exact incidence of fecal incontinence is unknown, and
a large portion of the suffering individuals probably does not seek medical
attention, due to embarrassment and unawareness of treatment options. In
most cases, however, quality of life can be significantly improved with adequate treatment, and new horizons in the treatment of fecal incontinence
have recently emerged.

Diagnosis and evaluation

Continence is a complex function of multiple factors working in concert,
including anatomic, physiologic, dietary, and psychological factors. Fecal
incontinence (FI) is the result of malfunction of one or more of the following mechanisms: colonic motility, stool consistency, anal sphincter structure
and function, rectal reservoir, anorectal sensory function, and pelvic floor
musculature and nerves. Patient evaluation should reveal the underlying
disturbed mechanisms.

History

A detailed bowel history is most important in evaluation of FI and its
impact on quality of life as expressed by a symptom score.[1] Symptom

diaries are probably the best way to monitor events. Urinary incontinence should be sought as there is a frequent coexistence with FI. A history of trauma or abdominal/pelvic/anal surgery as well as obstetric trauma in female subjects is essential. A detailed history of systemic diseases such as systemic sclerosis or multiple sclerosis should be achieved.

Physical examination

Careful examination can identify structural defects such as rectal mass, mucosal intussusception, prolapse, and rectocele. The perineal area should be inspected visually for excoriation, rash, scars, fistula opening, hemorrhoids, patulous anus, obvious cloacae, or 'keyhole deformity'. Perianal sensation is examined by local skin stimulation. Digital examination can provide an estimate of resting and squeeze tone of the anal sphincter, the existence of fecal impaction and pelvic floor descent. A bidigital examination may be performed to assess the integrity of the perineal body.

Anorectal manometry

The most widely used method to assess anal sphincter function is anorectal manometry[2] (Figure 14.1). Manometry provides information on resting and squeeze pressures, length of anal canal, and high-pressure zone. Resting pressure reflects mainly the internal anal sphincter (IAS) function, which comprises about 50–70% of anal tone. During examination, squeeze pressure as well as excitatory reflexes, which reflect external anal sphincter (EAS) function (e.g. cough reflex), can be elicited. Using a balloon attached to the tip of the catheter, rectoanal inhibitory reflex (RAIR), rectal sensory thresholds, and maximal rectal capacity can be assessed. Reservoir function of the rectum is an essential factor in continence mechanism, which results from the viscoelastic properties of the rectal wall, and enables low intraluminal pressure to be maintained while increasing rectal volume. Low rectal compliance may lead to decreased rectal capacity and, consequently, urgency and incontinence (e.g. proctitis).

Rectal sensation measured by balloon inflation is also an important factor in continence. Three basic thresholds are measured: first sensation, constant urge to defecate, and maximal tolerable capacity.

Endoanal ultrasound

The most valuable technique in assessing IAS and EAS defects is endoanal ultrasound. In experienced hands, sensitivity and specificity could reach nearly 100%. The endoprobe is inserted into the deep anal canal and pulled back. Images of the puborectalis muscle, anococcygeal ligament, perineal body, IAS, and EAS are seen (Figure 14.2). This examination has been regarded by some researchers as the study most likely to change patients' management.[3]

Magnetic resonance imaging

The pelvic floor can be visualized with an endorectal/endoanal coil. Magnetic resonance imaging (MRI) has a higher spatial resolution for imaging anal sphincters. Transverse planes are useful in diagnostics and surgery.

Electromyography

Concentric or single-fiber needle electromyography (EMG) is of importance for striated muscle sphincter mapping. This technique has been superseded by endoanal ultrasound for EAS and IAS defect assessment, as this examination is invasive, painful, and requires expertise. EMG is still the gold standard for functional innervation of the sphincter muscle.[4] The use of surface electrodes means that EMG can provide useful and painless information and has a definite role in applying biofeedback training.

(a)

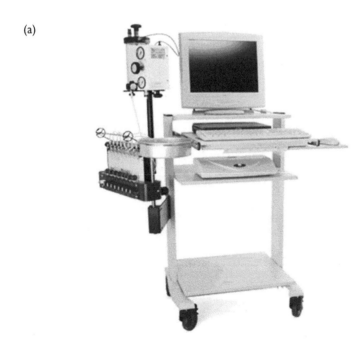

Figure 14.1 (a) The anal manometry system. Reproduction of this image courtesy of Medtronic.

(b)

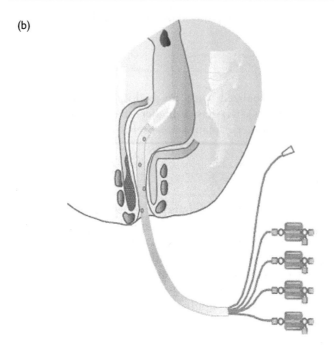

(c)

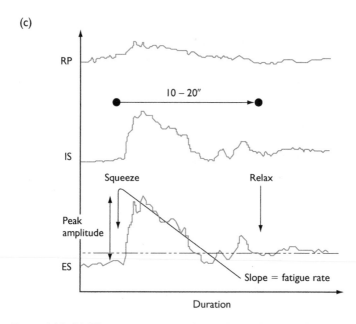

Figure 14.1 (b) The manometry catheter. Reproduction of this image courtesy of Medtronic. (c) Anal pressures.

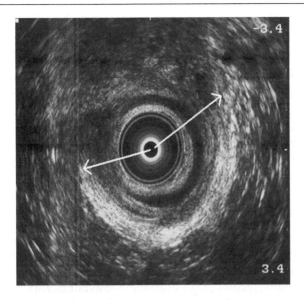

Figure 14.2 Anal ultrasound using a 7 MHz circular probe at the level of the middle anal canal, showing anterior defect at the internal and external sphincters (arrows at the defect edges) as a result of an obstetric injury.

Pudendal nerve terminal motor latency

The pudendal nerve contains motor fibers from sacral nerves S2–4 innervating the EAS and sensory innervation from the perineum. Pudendal nerve terminal motor latency (PNTML) measures conduction time from the distal part of this nerve to the EAS. In this technique, a flexible stimulatory electrode mounted on the examiner's hand is inserted into the anal canal. Electrical stimulation is given to the terminal branch of the nerve, and the time delay to contraction response of EAS is used to assess both left and right pudendal nerves.

Treatment modalities

Treatment options for fecal incontinence include conservative modalities such as biofeedback therapy, as well as minor surgical procedures and major surgery such as the neosphincter procedures. It is essential to carefully tailor the appropriate treatment to each patient, based on the severity of incontinence, work-up findings, past medical history, and the patient's wish.

Non-surgical methods

DIETARY MEASURES

Counseling the patient regarding diarrhea-inducing foods, possible sources of food intolerance, and addition of bulk-forming agents to the diet is often an initial step that can improve mild to moderate incontinence. The best method to pinpoint offending food is to use a daily food diary or systematic diet that eliminates potential offending agents. Gradual increase in dietary fiber up to 20–30 g/day increases stool bulk and may improve continence.

BOWEL MANAGEMENT

The goal of an effective bowel management program is to allow the patient to produce a bowel movement at a scheduled time using a combination of dietary measures, laxatives, suppositories, enemas, or digitation in order to achieve an 'empty rectum', thus enabling a few hours without the fear of incontinence episodes. This approach, mainly used by spinal cord injury patients, is also useful for patients with neurodegenerative diseases and congenital disorders.

ANTIDIARRHEALS

The most commonly used antidiarrheals are opium derivatives and absorbents such as loperamide. In addition to increasing colonic transit time, fluid absorption, and inhibition of mucus secretion, loperamide has also been found to increase anal sphincter tone.[5] A more potent derivative is diphenoxylate hydrochloride and tincture of opium. Low-dose tricyclic antidepressant (e.g. amitriptyline) offers improvement in FI due to anticholinergic and serotoninergic properties.

BIOFEEDBACK TRAINING

This term describes a therapeutic instrument from a psychological standpoint, and it has been found to be effective in therapy of FI. The anal sphincter function, which can be poorly perceived by the patient, is measured by a technical device and demonstrated ('feedback') to the subject, using a visual, auditory, or verbal signal (Figure 14.3). A common training program uses 30–60 minutes per session, at least once a week over a 6-week period. The mechanism of action is not entirely clear, and probably involves exercises to strengthen the EAS, enhancement of rectal sensitivity via an intrarectal balloon inflation, and improved coordination between rectal distention and sphincter contraction. Success rates vary in different series,

(a)

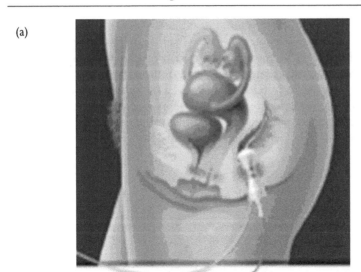

(b)

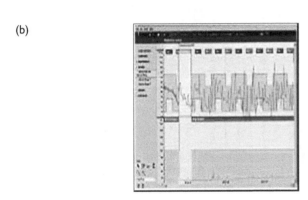

Figure 14.3 (a) Anal biofeedback probe. Reproduction of this image courtesy of Medtronic. (b) Feedback projected on the computer screen. Reproduction of this image courtesy of Medtronic.

reaching 64–89% of improvement.[6] Patients should have at least some rectal sensation as well as the ability to control sphincter contraction to fit for biofeedback, irrespective of the etiologies.

PROCON DEVICE

The ProCon is a soft catheter with a balloon, which can be inserted by the patient into the anal canal. When the balloon is inflated, it mechanically obstructs the anal canal, preventing fecal leakage. The catheter tip is equipped with an infrared photo-interrupter sensor, connected to a beeper-like monitor (Fig 14.4). Whenever fecal content reaches the anal canal, the beeper goes off, and the patient may go to the bathroom, deflate the balloon, and evacuate. An initial study[7] showed that although only some of the patients tolerated the device, these patients had significant improvement in their continence score. New versions of the device are now under development and may be better tolerated by the patients.

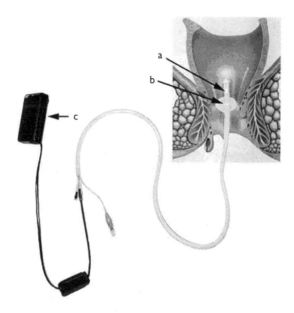

Figure 14.4 (a) The ProCon device: double-lumen, pliable rubber catheter. The distal tip incorporates an infrared photo-interrupter sensor and flatus vent holes. (b) Inflatable 20 ml capacity cuff. (c) Monitor, resembling a common beeper.

Surgical methods

ANTERIOR SPHINCTER REPAIR

Obstetric injury causing anterior defect of the external anal sphincter at the rectovaginal septum is the most common cause of fecal incontinence, and may be clinically evident only years after vaginal delivery. When anterior sphincter defect is detected by anal ultrasound, and innervation of the sphincter mechanism is intact, sphincter repair is probably the surgical treatment of choice.

The surgical procedure usually involves mobilization of the external anal sphincter on both sides. When damage exists, the anterior portion of the sphincter usually consists of a fibrotic scar, which is divided. The muscle from both sides is then approximated, with overlap of one side on the other, using nonabsorbable sutures (Figure 14.5).

The short-term success rate is high, with significant improvement in continence and quality of life, and may nearly reach 80%.[8] However, recent data suggest that the long-term success rate may be lower, and durable continence may be achieved in approximately 45% of patients.[9]

INTERNAL SPHINCTER BULKING PROCEDURES

Several procedures are aimed to increase the internal anal sphincter bulk in order to improve anal resting pressure. The *Acyst procedure* uses carbon-coated beads, which may be injected into the internal sphincter as an office procedure. The procedure is simple and safe, and preliminary reports have shown some improvement in continence.[10] Injection of silicon particles resulted in similar results.

The *Secca procedure* uses thermal energy to create scarring and fibrosis of the internal anal sphincter, using the same technology as for the Stretta procedure of the lower gastroesophageal sphincter. The device is inserted

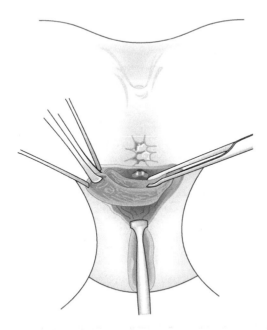

Figure 14.5 Anterior sphincter repair. The patient is in the prone position.

into the anal canal, and needles are introduced into the internal sphincter muscle to deliver the thermal energy under continuous monitoring (Figure 14.6). The Secca procedure may be performed as an office procedure under local anesthesia and mild sedation, without major side-effects, and preliminary results suggest improvement in continence and quality of life.[11]

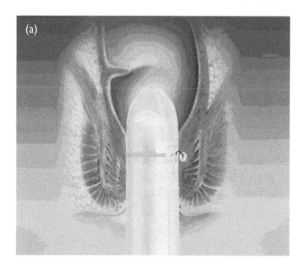

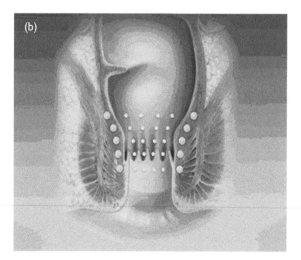

Figure 14.6 (a, b) The Secca procedure. Reproduced with permission from Curon Medical, Inc.

SACRAL NERVE STIMULATION

Sensory, autonomic, and motor innervation of the pelvic floor organs are all mediated by the sacral nerves. Continuous electrical stimulation of the sacral roots was found to improve pelvic floor function, including fecal incontinence. The exact mechanism of effect is not clear, but it is assumed that both enhanced sensation and augmentation of the motor signal play a role in this procedure. Sacral nerve stimulation uses leads connected to a stimulator for electric stimulation of the sacral nerve roots (Figure 14.7). The leads are stimulated intraoperatively, to determine the roots with the best motor external anal sphincter response. The leads with the best response are then connected to a temporary external stimulator, for a test stimulation period of 3 weeks, in which the patient fills a daily continence diary. If there is significant improvement, a permanent pacemaker is implanted in the subcutaneous tissue. Preliminary results are encouraging, suggesting that 75–100% of the implanted patients experienced improved continence, and 41–75% achieved complete continence.[12] However, larger series and longer follow-up are required to determine the role of this procedure in the treatment of fecal incontinence.

NEOSPHINCTER PROCEDURES – STIMULATED GRACILIS

In the case of 'end-stage' fecal incontinence, not manageable by primary surgical repair, the construction of a new nonanatomic sphincter may be

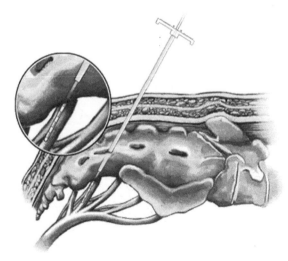

Figure 14.7 Sacral nerve stimulation. Reproduction of this image courtesy of Medtronic.

required. Several muscle flaps were offered for anal neosphincter procedures, but the gracilis muscle transposition is by far the most commonly
used flap. The gracilis muscle originates at the inferior border of the pubis,
and crosses the medial aspect of the thigh to its insertion at the medial
aspect of the proximal tibia. The muscle is divided distally at its insertion
and dissected free of the thigh structures in the proximal direction through
three small thigh incisions. The neurovascular bundle supplying the gracilis
muscle enters near its origin, allowing the rotation of this long muscle to the
perianal region to wrap it around the anal canal, and anchor to the ischial
bone (Figure 14.8). Although this procedure can improve basal anal tone,
the gracilis is a skeletal muscle which cannot maintain sustained contraction, resulting in muscle fatigue. The stimulated gracilis procedure uses an
electric stimulator at the entrance of the neurovascular bundle to stimulate
the gracilis muscle continuously. This continuous electric stimulation results
in transformation of the gracilis muscle to a nonfatigable muscle, and the
stimulation can be modified or switched off as needed. Despite its complexity, about 60% of patients experience significant improvement in
continence.[13]

ARTIFICIAL BOWEL SPHINCTER

The artificial bowel sphincter (ABS) is a silicone inflatable implant that
aims to produce a controllable continuous anal tone. The device has three
main components:

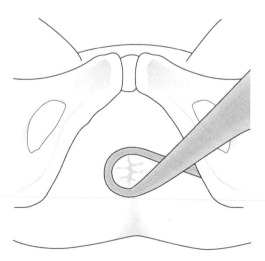

Figure 14.8 Gracilis transposition neosphincter. The patient is in the lithotomy position.

- the inflatable cuff is implanted around the anal canal, and, when inflated, produces the basal pressure;
- the pressurized balloon is a reservoir implanted at the lower abdominal wall behind the pubic bone;
- the pump, which is implanted in the scrotum in males, and in the labia in females, allows the patient to control the shift of fluids between the cuff and the balloon.

When the patient wishes to evacuate, he or she presses the pump, which mechanically shifts fluid from the cuff to the balloon. The cuff spontaneously reinflates within a few minutes, re-establishing anal tone (Figure 14.9).

As expected, a silicone implant around the anus carries a high rate of infectious complications, frequently requiring removal or revision of the device. Other frequent complications include cuff erosion and device failure. Despite these drawbacks, this procedure is simpler than the muscle neosphincter procedures such as the stimulated gracilis, and is gaining increased popularity. A multicenter study of 112 patients in 19 centers revealed that 71% of the patients had a functioning device 1 year postimplantation, with a significant improvement in continence and quality of

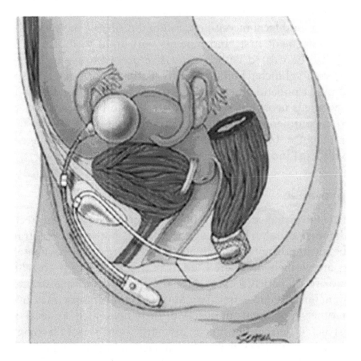

Figure 14.9 Artificial bowel sphincter in a female. Acticon Neosphincter. Courtesy of American Medical Systems, Inc., Minnetonka, MN.

life,[14] and recent single-center experience of 37 patients showed that the success rate further improves with more experience.[15]

STOMA CREATION

Creation of a stoma is usually regarded as the last option for the treatment of fecal incontinence, and is usually saved for patients who have failed multiple treatments. However, in elderly and high-risk patients, and in patients unwilling to undergo complicated procedures and their associated risks, a stoma may be considered at an earlier stage. Temporary diversion may also be considered to protect complicated procedures, and to improve quality of life until healing is complete, although no data to support this approach are available.

Clinical approach to patient with fecal incontinence

Fecal incontinence interferes with quality of life, and its treatment needs to be tailored to the patients' needs. Although it is tough to outline a strict flow chart that will be accepted by all experts, the choice of treatment should be guided by the severity of incontinence and its effect on quality of life, and results of the anatomic and physiologic work-up.

Patients with mild fecal incontinence should probably have a trial of non-operative management first, and patients with mild to moderate incontinence may also be treated with less-invasive procedures such as the Secca and the internal sphincter bulking agents. Patients with external sphincter injury and intact pudendal nerves will probably be best treated with surgical repair, whereas neosphincter procedures should be reserved for patients with severe incontinence that cannot be primarily restored, or in failure of such repair. Figure 14.10 suggests a flow chart for the management of patients with fecal incontinence.

Rectal prolapse

Complete rectal prolapse is a full-thickness protrusion of the rectal wall through the anal canal. The etiology is unclear, but increased straining is likely to be an important cause. In Western countries approximately 80% of patients are women and there is an increased incidence in the elderly.

The majority of patients experience the prolapse during strain, which may spontaneously reduce after defecation. Rectal prolapse may be associated with other functional anorectal disturbances such as fecal incontinence, obstructed defecation, mucus discharge, and rectal bleeding. When fecal incontinence is associated with damaged sphincter or pudendal neuropathy, repair of the prolapse may not improve continence. Constipation

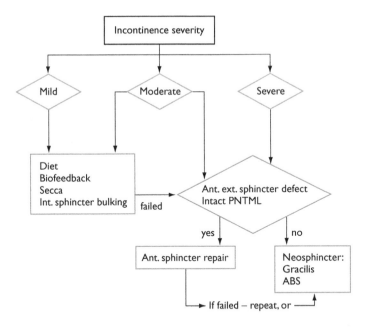

Figure 14.10 Suggested flowchart for the management of patients with fecal incontinence.

may improve, remain unchanged, or even worsen by the repair, depending on the reason for the constipation and the surgical technique.

Inspecting the perineum while asking the patient to strain usually makes the diagnosis. If unsuccessful on the examination bed, the patient may be asked to strain in the sitting position. Examination may also reveal patulous anal orifice with lax sphincters and excoriation of the perianal skin. Other tests may include anorectal physiology tests, constipation work-up if necessary, and colonoscopy to exclude coexisting pathology.

Treatment

The principal treatment of rectal prolapse is surgical, aimed at selecting the procedure with minimal morbidity and the lowest recurrence rate. Procedures for the correction of prolapse can be broadly divided into two large categories, abdominal and perineal.

Abdominal procedures

Abdominal repairs require laparotomy or laparoscopy under general anesthesia to access the peritoneal cavity. These operations may be categorized into rectopexy alone with or without mesh, resection with rectopexy, and resection alone.

SUTURE RECTOPEXY

All abdominal procedures imply pelvic dissection with rectal mobilization. The sigmoid colon and rectum are mobilized, taking care to identify the left ureter and the hypogastric nerves. Anteriorly, the rectum is mobilized to the upper end of the vagina, and posteriorly, the presacral space is entered in front of the presacral nerves and dissected to the level of the tip of the coccyx. Controversy exists as to the need for lateral mobilization of the rectum. The rectum is then pulled up to reduce the prolapse, and secured to the sacrum by sutures.

Simple suture rectopexy effectively repairs rectal prolapse, with recurrence rate averaging 3–7%.[16] Since there is no anastomosis, the operation carries minimal risk of sepsis. However, constipation is usually not improved, and patients not constipated preoperatively may become so following this procedure.[17]

POSTERIOR RECTOPEXY WITH FOREIGN MATERIAL

These procedures use a foreign material to fix the prolapsed rectum to the sacrum. The rectum and the sigmoid colon are mobilized as described above. Then a sheet of artificial material such as Ivalon sponge, Vicryl mesh, or Marlex mesh is fixed to the sacrum using interrupted 2-0 Prolene sutures. The 'wings' of the artificial material are attached to the sides of the rectum, not wrapping it completely (Figure 14.11). Reported recurrence rates may be somewhat lower than with rectopexy alone.[18] However, postoperative constipation is common, and may be disabling.[19]

RESECTION RECTOPEXY

The combination of rectopexy and resection of the sigmoid colon was popularized by Frykman and Goldberg. The pelvic dissection is performed as described, and the resection is identical to high anterior resection, with the addition of sutured rectopexy to the presacral fascia (Figure 14.12). This procedure is probably associated with the lowest recurrence rate, averaging 3–4% (range 1–10%), and a decreased incidence of debilitating constipation.[20] However, since the procedure involves resection with a colorectal anastomosis, it carries the highest risk of septic complications, with associated morbidity and possible mortality.

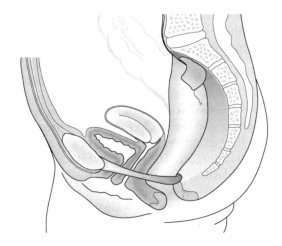

Figure 14.11 Mesh rectopexy.

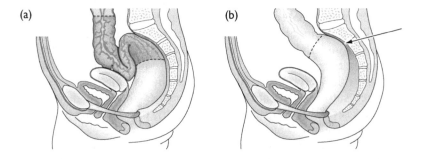

Figure 14.12 (a) The resected segment of a resection rectopexy. (b) Anastomosis and rectopexy. An arrow points to the sutures attaching the upper rectum to the sacrum.

Laparoscopic approach

Laparoscopic rectopexy was first reported in 1993. The patient is placed supine in the Lloyd-Davies Trendelenburg position and 3–4 ports are placed. The abdominal cavity is insufflated with CO_2, and the camera is usually introduced through the umbilical port. Rectal mobilization to the pelvic floor and rectal fixation to the sacrum with or without resection use the same principles described for the open procedure. Fixation to the sacrum by sutures or mesh can be laparoscopically achieved.

Reported recurrence rates are acceptable, but long-term results are still to be evaluated. Short-term advantages include less pain, shorter hospitalization, early return of bowel function, and faster recovery.[21]

Perineal procedures

Perineal operations are attractive as they can be applied in sick, elderly, or high-risk patients safely, without the use of general anesthesia. In addition, in young male patients they avoid the risk to sexual and bladder dysfunction associated with pelvic surgery. However, the main drawback of the perineal approach is the relatively high recurrence rate compared with the abdominal procedures.[22]

As with abdominal operations, there is a wide variety of perineal operations of which mucosal sleeve resection (Delorme's operation) and perineal rectosigmoidectomy (Altmeier's operation) are the most commonly used.

DELORME'S OPERATION

The procedure may be carried out in the lithotomy or prone jackknife position. The rectum is prolapsed to its full extent. The mucosa is incised circumferentially 1–2 cm above the dentate line, and a mucosal tube is dissected off the underlying muscle in the proximal direction. Once the dissection reaches the apex of the prolapse, the mucosal tube is excised. Several absorbable Vicryl sutures are placed circumferentially to plicate the prolapse. Each suture begins at the divided mucosa above the dentate line and then takes several bites of muscle proximally, to end at the mucosa at the apex of the prolapse (Figure 14.13).

Mucosal sleeve resection has gained popularity in the last few years owing to its low morbidity. Since there is no full-thickness resection and anastomosis, the risk of pelvic sepsis is minimal. However, this procedure is probably associated with the highest recurrence rate, averaging 12–15%.[23]

ALTMEIER'S OPERATION

This procedure may be carried out in the lithotomy or prone jackknife position. After the prolapse has been delivered, a circumferential incision is made through the full thickness of the rectal wall 2 cm above the dentate line. The rectum is drawn down to expose the peritoneal reflection anteriorly, which is incised to enter the peritoneal cavity. Once the peritoneal cavity has been exposed, the rectum and sigmoid are drawn down as far as possible. The mesentery is ligated and divided close to the bowel wall until the bowel cannot be prolapsed further. The sigmoid colon is divided and the proximal sigmoid is anastomosed to the anal canal using interrupted Vicryl sutures or a circular stapler.

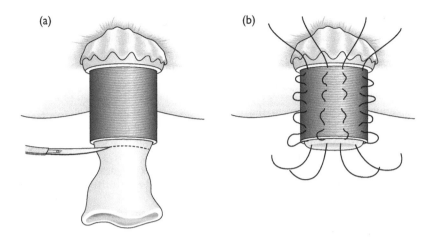

Figure 14.13 (a) Resection of the mucosal sleeve in a Delorme's procedure. (b) Plication of the muscular coat in a Delorme's procedure.

Perineal rectosigmoidectomy is simple, effective, and well tolerated even by high-risk patients. Recurrence rates are higher than for abdominal repair, averaging 10%, but are probably lower in comparison to the mucosal sleeve resection.[24] Main complications include bleeding and anastomotic dehiscence with a potential pelvic sepsis.

Selection of operative procedure

A uniformed surgical operation is not appropriate for all patients with rectal prolapse, and the appropriate procedure should be tailored to each patient's need, based on the integration of the operative risk, recurrence rate, and functional results.[25] There is no doubt that a perineal procedure is associated with less morbidity than abdominal procedures. Old or unfit patients are probably best treated with the perineal procedures. A perineal rectosigmoidectomy may be preferred if the prolapse is large. Smaller prolapses may be best treated with a Delorme's procedure.

Abdominal procedures should usually be considered in young and fit females with rectal prolapse; however, the specific choice of procedure is more controversial. For patients without constipation, rectopexy alone should be sufficient, since the recurrence rate is low and restoration of continence is similar for all abdominal procedures. For patients with significant constipation, resection rectopexy results in good functional results with decreased incidence of constipation.

References

1. Jorge JM, Wexner SD. Etiology and management of fecal incontinence. Dis Col Rectum 1993;36:77–97.
2. Azpiroz F, Enck P, Whitehead WE. Anorectal function testing: review of collective experience. Am J Gastroenterol 2002;97:232–40.
3. Liberman H, Faria J, Ternent CA, et al. A prospective evaluation of the value of anorectal physiology in the management of fecal incontinence. Dis Col Rectum 2001;44:1567–74.
4. Cheong DM, Vaccaro CA, Salanga VD. Electrodiagnostic evaluation of fecal incontinence. Muscle Nerve 1995;18:612–19.
5. Read M, Read NW, Barber DC, et al. Effects of loperamide on anal sphincter function in patients complaining of chronic diarrhea with fecal incontinence and urgency. Dig Dis Sci 1982;27:807–14.
6. Ozturck R, Niazi S, Stessman M, Rao SSC. Long-term outcome and objective changes in anorectal function after biofeedback therapy for fecal incontinence. Aliment Pharmacol Ther 2004;20:667–74.
7. Giamundo P, Welber A, Weiss EG, et al. The procon incontinence device: a new nonsurgical approach to preventing episodes of fecal incontinence. Am J Gastroenterol 2002;97(9):2328–32.
8. Rothbarth J, Bemelman WA, Meijerink WJ, et al. Long-term results of anterior anal sphincter repair for fecal incontinence due to obstetric injury/with invited commentaries. Dig Surg 2000;17(4):390–3.
9. Halverson AL, Hull TL. Long-term outcome of overlapping anal sphincter repair. Dis Colon Rectum 2002;45(3):345–8.
10. Weiss E, Efron J, Nogueras J, Wexner S. Submucosal injection of carbon coated beads is a successful and safe office-based treatment of fecal incontinence. Dis Colon Rectum 2002;45:46–7.
11. Efron JE, Corman ML, Fleshman J, et al. Safety and effectiveness of temperature-controlled radio-frequency energy delivery to the anal canal (Secca procedure) for the treatment of fecal incontinence. Dis Colon Rectum 2003;46(12):1606–16.
12. Jarrett ME, Mowatt G, Glazener CM, et al. Systematic review of sacral nerve stimulation for faecal incontinence and constipation. Br J Surg 2004; 91(12):1559–69.
13. Wexner SD, Baeten C, Bailey R, et al. Long-term efficacy of dynamic gracilo-plasty for fecal incontinence. Dis Colon Rectum 2002;45(6):809–18.
14. Wong WD, Congliosi SM, Spencer MP, et al. The safety and efficacy of the artificial bowel sphincter for fecal incontinence: results from a multicenter cohort study. Dis Colon Rectum 2002;45(9):1139–53.
15. Michot F, Costaglioli B, Leroi AM, Denis P. Artificial anal sphincter in severe fecal incontinence: outcome of prospective experience with 37 patients in one institution. Ann Surg 2003;237(1):52–6.
16. Novell JR, Osborne MJ, Winslet MC, Lewis AA. Prospective randomized trial of Ivalon sponge versus sutured rectopexy for full-thickness rectal prolapse. Br J Surg 1994;81(6):904–6.
17. Madden MV, Kamm MA, Nicholls RJ, et al. Abdominal rectopexy for complete prolapse: prospective study evaluating changes in symptoms and anorectal function. Dis Colon Rectum 1992;35:48–55.

18. Keighley MR, Fielding JW, Alexander-Williams J. Results of Marlex mesh abdominal rectopexy for rectal prolapse in 100 consecutive patients. Br J Surg 1983;70:229–32

19. Mann CV, Hoffman C. Complete rectal prolapse: the anatomical and functional results of treatment by an extended abdominal rectopexy. Br J Surg 1988;75:34–7.

20. McKee RF, Lauder JC, Poon FW, Aitchison MA, Finlay IG. A prospective randomised study of abdominal rectopexy with and without sigmoidectomy in rectal prolapse. Surg Gynecol Obstet 1992;174:145–8.

21. Solomon MJ, Young CJ, Eyers AA, Roberts RA. Randomized clinical trial of laparoscopic versus open abdominal rectopexy for rectal prolapse. Br J Surg 2002;89:35–9.

22. Watts JD, Rothenberger DA, Buls JG, Goldberg SM, Nivatvongs S. The management of procidentia: 30 years experience. Dis Colon Rectum 1985; 28:96–102.

23. Watts AM, Thompson MR. Evaluation of Delorme's procedure as a treatment for full-thickness rectal prolapse. Br J Surg 2000;87:218–22.

24. Azimuddin K, Khubchandani IT, Rosen L, et al. Rectal prolapse: a search for the 'best' operation. Am Surg 2001;67:622–7.

25. Brown AJ, Anderson JH, McKee RF, Finlay IG. Strategy for selection of type of operation for rectal prolapse based on clinical criteria. Dis Colon Rectum 2004;47:103–7.

Chapter 15

Female sexual dysfunction: current management

Lawrence S Hakim

Introduction

Since the release of sildenafil (Viagra, Pfizer) for the treatment of male erectile dysfunction or ED, in 1998, there has been a significant increase in the amount of public and media attention focused on the topic of 'female sexual dysfunction' or FSD. In fact, more and more, the medical community and women in general are beginning to understand that FSD may, in part, be due to 'physical' or organic issues, and not purely psychologic or psychosexual in nature, as many previously believed. This new understanding has also led to the development of various effective treatment options, which are now available to help women and couples improve their sexual health.

In this chapter we will explore the demographics and causative factors associated with FSD, as well as the basic work-up of these women. Current management alternatives will also be discussed.

Demographics of female sexual dysfunction: the epidemic

In 2001, a demographic study in the *Journal of the American Medical Association (JAMA)* demonstrated that more than 40% of women had evidence of FSD. Based on population surveys, this would suggest that more than 30 million women in the USA might have female sexual dysfunction. Unfortunately, due to a number of factors, currently less than 3% of women with FSD seek help. Some of the factors responsible for this include the fact that the majority of women are not routinely, if ever, asked about the presence of sexual dysfunction by their physician. Like ED, many women are embarrassed to bring up the topic and it goes unnoticed. Additionally, many women have no idea that there are effective treatment options available once the problem has been identified by their healthcare professional.

Why is this a problem? Because normal sexual function is an important part of the 'essential intimacy' between a woman and her partner ('the *couple*'). The loss of sexual function may lead to loss of self-esteem, guilt, depression, and alienation from one's partner. Like erectile dysfunction in men, FSD is a *spectrum* of disease, not necessarily an 'all or none' phenomenon, and should be identified and treated even in its earliest stages.

A key point to remember is that like ED, its counterpart in the male, FSD may be an early warning sign of significant unrecognized systemic vascular disease and indicate an increased risk for heart attack or stroke. Epidemiologic studies noted an increased risk of FSD in women with a history of common vascular risk factors, such as cigarette smoking, hypercholesterolemia, hypertension, and prior hysterectomy. Therefore, it is critical for the healthcare professional to 'ask the question' and to recognize FSD early and encourage communication between the patient and her partner.

The female sexual response

The female sexual response was studied and described by Masters and Johnson in the 1960s. They divided it into four stages: excitement, plateau, orgasm, and resolution. In 1979, Helen Singer Kaplan proposed a triphasic response: desire, arousal, and orgasm. In 2001, Dr Rosemary Basson[1] proposed a 'non-linear' female sexual response cycle (Figure 15.1). She suggested that the sexual response is driven by the *desire to enhance intimacy*. The cycle begins with *sexual neutrality*. As a woman seeks a sexual stimulus and responds to it, she becomes sexually aroused. Arousal leads to desire, thus stimulating a woman's willingness to receive or provide additional stimuli. Emotional and physical satisfactions are gained by an increase in sexual desire and arousal. Emotional intimacy is then ultimately achieved. Various biologic and psychologic factors can negatively affect this cycle, thus leading to FSD.

Physiology of female sexual function

Clitoral and labial vascular engorgement is similar to engorgement of the corpora cavernosa in the male during erection. Vaginal lubrication is in many ways analogous to penile erection in the male, in that adequate vascular function plays a critical role. Recent studies have demonstrated an important role for androgens and nitric oxide in the mechanism of genital vascular engorgement during the female sexual response. It is this fact that has led to the introduction of hormone replacement therapy (HRT) and various oral medications, most notably the PDE5 (phosphodiesterase type 5) inhibitors such as sildenafil, as treatment options for sexual arousal insufficiency and other forms of FSD.

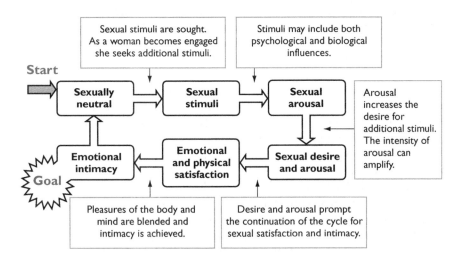

Figure 15.1 Female sexual response cycle. Reproduced from Basson R. Human sex-response cycles. J Sex Marital Ther 2001;27:33–43.

Classification of female sexual dysfunction

There are many different categories of sexual dysfunction in women, as there are in men. Female sexual dysfunction can be classified into

- sexual desire disorders
- sexual arousal disorders
- orgasmic disorders
- sexual pain disorders.

Dysfunctions of the desire phase (as defined in the DSM-IV) include hypoactive sexual desire disorder and sexual aversion disorder.

Dysfunctions of the arousal phase include female sexual arousal disorder, as well as vaginismus and dyspareunia. Orgasm phase disorders include female orgasmic disorder. Overlap between symptoms is often seen.

Risk factors for female sexual dysfunction

Female sexual dysfunction can occur at any age and numerous risk factors can be implicated as contributing to the development of FSD. These can be broken up into hormonal or endocrine disorders, vascular factors, neurologic issues, medications, gynecologic disorders, psychogenic causes, and factors associated with aging.

Endocrinologic changes are among the most common causative factors in women suffering from sexual dysfunction. Androgen insufficiency syndrome may occur when the androgen levels required for the normal sexual response and normal libido are abnormally low.

Postmenopausal hormone changes, such as diminished local or systemic estrogen levels, can also contribute to FSD. Other endocrinologic factors associated with FSD include hypothyroidism, hyperthyroidism, pituitary tumors, and hyperprolactinemia.

Genital blood flow is critical to the normal female sexual response and various vasculopathies can contribute to sexual dysfunction. These may include atherosclerosis and its associated risk factors, smoking, diabetes, dyslipidemia, peripheral vascular disease, hypertension, pelvic and perineal trauma, and arterial compression from cycling.

There are numerous gynecologic etiologies of female sexual dysfunction, as listed in Table 15.1. These can be differentiated into external or internal abnormalities. All should be considered during the comprehensive physical evaluation. Certain medications and drugs may be associated with female sexual dysfunction. Some of these agents are listed in Table 15.2.

Table 15.1 Gynecologic etiologies of female sexual dysfunction

External	Internal
Vulvar dystrophy	Vaginismus
Dermatitis	Vaginal tissue atrophy
Clitoral adhesions	Vaginitis
Clitoral phimosis	Uterine prolapse
Bartholin's cysts	Cystocele/rectocele
Episiotomy scars	Pelvic inflammatory disease
Vestibulitis	Uterine fibroids
Vulvar cancer	Endometriosis
Lichen sclerosus	Myalgias
	Cancer

Table 15.2 Drugs associated with female sexual dysfunction

Antidepressants	Psychotropics
Antihypertensives	Beta-blockers
Narcotics	Cocaine, alcohol
Diuretics	Lipid-lowering drugs
Antiandrogens	NSAIDs
H₂ blockers	Oncologic agents
Anticholinergics	Anxiolytics

Neurogenic causes of FSD are not uncommon and may be associated with neurologic disease or surgery. Some of the causes include:

- radical pelvic surgery, such as colorectal surgery and radical hysterectomy
- pelvic and spinal cord injury
- multiple sclerosis
- various neuropathies
- pudendal nerve injury
- stroke
- Alzheimer's disease
- Parkinson's disease.

Female sexual dysfunction can occur at any age, and unlike ED in men, it is as often seen in young, sexually active women as it is in older women. However, there is a significant association between sexual dysfunction and aging due to numerous age-associated changes. These include a progressive decline in physiologic function, genital and vaginal atrophy, decreased vaginal lubrication, the increased prevalence of chronic diseases, as well as various psychologic issues and partner issues commonly seen in the elderly. However, decreased sexual activity does not have to be inevitable with aging.

There are various psychogenic causes that are associated with sexual dysfunction. Some of the more common factors are depression, performance anxiety, relationship problems, psychosocial problems, and psychologic distress.

Diagnostic evaluation of female sexual dysfunction

A 'step-care' approach to FSD management has been demonstrated to be an effective means of evaluating and successfully managing women who are experiencing sexual dysfunction. Excellent communication with the partner and physician is the first step in this approach. It is important to identify reversible causes, such as smoking or various medications – i.e. SSRIs (selective serotonin reuptake inhibitors) – that may be contributing to FSD, and institute healthy lifestyle changes. It is critical to evaluate the woman completely to understand 'why' the problem exists, since FSD, like ED in the male, may be the *first* sign of other underlying disease, such as vascular disease, lipid disorder or diabetes. Remembering the word 'I.N.T.I.M.A.C.Y.', which is further described in Table 15.3, can summarize the eight basic steps in the management of FSD.

Female sexual dysfunction is evaluated like any other disease. The first step, a complete medical and sexual history, is important to define the problem. This will allow the physician to identify the various risk factors, which were previously described. In addition, any history of abuse is important to elicit. It is important to define or classify the type of dysfunction, since effective treatment strategies will vary based on the diagnosis. There are various validated questionnaires, such as the 'FSFI' or Female Sexual Function Index, that can be utilized to objectively define and monitor the FSD over time. A directed physical examination is also important as part of the initial evaluation. Documentation of a recent normal PAP smear and breast examination should be made, or performed if not recently done. Various physical anatomic abnormalities, such as vaginal atrophy or clitoral phimosis (Figure 15.2), may contribute to FSD when present, and therefore need to be evaluated.

Table 15.3 I.N.T.I.M.A.C.Y.

I:	Identification
N:	Notification
T:	Thorough evaluation
I:	Incorporate lifestyle changes
M:	Medical and surgical therapy
A:	Alternative therapies
C:	Communication
Y:	Youthful rejuvenation

(a)

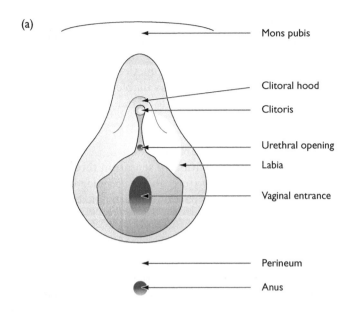

Mons pubis

Clitoral hood

Clitoris

Urethral opening

Labia

Vaginal entrance

Perineum

Anus

(b)

Normal   **Clitoral phimosis**

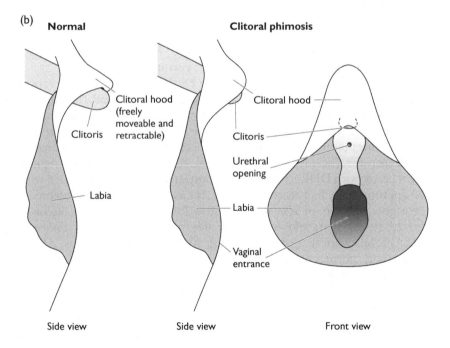

Clitoral hood
(freely
moveable and
retractable)

Clitoris

Labia

Clitoral hood

Clitoris

Urethral
opening

Labia

Vaginal
entrance

Side view   Side view   Front view

Figure 15.2 (a) Female genital anatomy. (b) Anatomic abnormalities may possibly contribute to sexual dysfunction.

As part of the comprehensive evaluation, selected laboratory studies should be obtained, including androgen levels, such as serum testosterone levels (total/free), dehydroepiandrosterone and its sulfate (DHEA/DHEA-S), sex hormone-binding globulin (SHBG), estradiol, a lipid panel, serum glucose, urinalysis, liver function studies, and thyroid function tests.

A number of specialized diagnostic tools available at certain tertiary centers can be used in specific circumstances to better define the FSD. They include:

- vaginal pH testing (as a gauge of arousal)
- biothesiometry (neurologic evaluation of sensation thresholds)
- duplex Doppler ultrasonography (to evaluate vascular function)
- temperature sensation testing (as part of a neurologic evaluation).

Treatment options

Once the diagnostic evaluation is completed, the next step is to discuss the various treatment options available for the patient. Some of the more simple options include a discussion of reversible and lifestyle changes. Patients should be instructed to give up or decrease smoking, and drinking in moderation should be encouraged. A healthy diet, with lowering of an elevated cholesterol, should be discussed if appropriate. Since anxiety and stress can worsen any type of sexual dysfunction, regular exercise and stress-reduction techniques should be discussed. Most importantly, good communication with the partner should be encouraged.

There are data to suggest that FSD can be effectively treated by various medical therapies. These may include androgen replacement therapy with DHEA and/or topical testosterone therapy, off-label PDE5 inhibitor drugs, and others. The role of newer therapeutic oral agents such as apomorphine, and other intranasal and topical agents are currently being investigated.

Androgen insufficiency is a major cause of FSD and hormone replacement therapy with DHEA has been demonstrated to be quite effective when used appropriately. In a recent study by Akkus and associates, presented at the European Society of Sexual Medicine in 2003, 55 women ranging in age from 23 to 54 years old (mean age: 43) with FSD and low androgen (DHEA) levels were treated with DHEA 50 mg/day for 3 months. All had partners with normal erectile function. At the completion of the study, all of the patients demonstrated increased DHEA levels and all of the women demonstrated objective improvement in the areas of desire (libido), arousal, and orgasm.

Sildenafil citrate (Viagra, Pfizer) and various other PDE5 inhibitors have been proven to be effective for male sexual dysfunction (ED), but are they effective in women? In a recent study, Berman et al[2] evaluated the efficacy and safety of sildenafil citrate in spontaneously or surgically postmenopausal women with female sexual arousal disorder (FSAD). All of the women had protocol-specified estradiol and free testosterone concentrations and/or were receiving estrogen and/or androgen replacement therapy to eliminate any androgen insufficiency. It was found that in women with FSAD, without concomitant hypoactive sexual desire disorder, sildenafil was associated with significantly greater improvement in sexual function than placebo.

It is important not to misdiagnose women suffering from FSD with depression, since many of the symptoms may be the same. Additionally, it has been shown that FSD may be worsened by the use of various antidepressant agents, including the SSRIs, such as Zoloft (sertraline), Paxil (paroxetine) and Prozac (fluoxetine). Due to the ultimate effects of these agents on the orgasm centers of the brain, the time to orgasm can be significantly delayed or worse (anorgasmia). For those women who need to continue antidepressant therapy in the face of FSD, buproprion (Welbutrin) is an agent often with less sexual side-effects than the SSRIs and it may be an effective alternative. In addition, various researchers have demonstrated that women taking SSRIs may benefit from the off-label use of PDE5 inhibitors such as sildenafil, to improve their sexual function, assuring first that there are no contraindications such as nitrate use or chance of pregnancy.

Specific therapies

In addition to safe and effective medical therapies for female sexual dysfunction, there are various 'specific' therapies that are useful in certain situations. As shown in Figure15.2b, clitoral phimosis is an anatomic anomaly that can contribute to orgasmic dysfunction and FSD. In many cases of minimal to moderate phimosis, topical estrogen therapy may be an effective first-line treatment option. For women with severe phimosis not responsive to topical therapy, there may be a role for surgical management.

After episiotomy, vaginal delivery, genital or pelvic surgery or trauma, the presence of neuromas or scar tissue can lead to sexual pain disorders and FSD. First-line therapy should include a minimally invasive approach, such as topical therapy or using a course of directed injections with a combination of steroid/local anesthetic. If this fails to improve the situation, there may be a role for surgery to remove the offending neuroma or scar.

EROS-clitoral therapy device

Currently, the only FDA-approved therapy for the treatment of female sexual dysfunction is the EROS-CTD (clitoral therapy device) illustrated in Figure 15.3. The EROS-CTD is a small, battery-powered, hand-held clitoral vacuum device, which, when applied to the genitalia, enhances clitoral

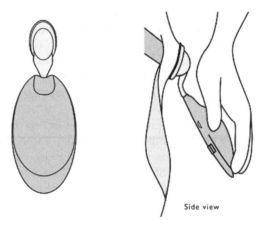

Side view

Figure 15.3 EROS-CTD (clitoral therapy device).

engorgement, increases clitoral blood flow, and improves arousal. Women have reported that the EROS-CTD device can improve genital sensation, increase vaginal lubrication, and improve the ability to achieve orgasm, leading to enhanced sexual satisfaction.

Role of sex therapy

Although many women with sexual dysfunction may have contributing physical or organic factors, there are certainly a number of psychologic and relationship issues that can also play a critical role in their FSD and need to be addressed at the same time. It has been shown that sex therapy by a licensed and certified professional can be very effective in helping a woman to overcome her FSD. However, although sex therapy is certainly noninvasive, it is important to remember that it may be time-consuming, and certainly requires 'commitment' on the part of the woman, and often her partner, too. Various other noninvasive techniques, such as pelvic floor exercises and biofeedback, can also be important adjuncts to successful therapy.

Sexual dysfunction is a couple's disease

It is imperative to remember that sexual dysfunction is a couple's disease! Whereas up to 43% of women between the ages of 18 and 59 years old may suffer from FSD (JAMA, 2001), 52% of men between the ages of 40 and 70 years old have ED (Feldman and associates, Massachusetts Male

Aging Study, 1994). For this reason, it is important to always involve the partner whenever possible in the diagnostic and treatment phases: otherwise, you're missing half of the equation! By involving the partner from the earliest stages, the couple can understand the underlying cause of the FSD, improve communication, avoid 'blame', identify and treat any sexual dysfunction in themselves and their partner, and help find a solution that works for both of them.

By understanding that no single treatment is right for everyone or every couple, and in order to accomplish the lofty goal of improving the woman's sexual dysfunction and the couple's intimacy, an individualized, multidisciplinary approach, involving the urologist, gynecologist, sex therapist, and primary care physician is ideal.

References

1. Basson R. Human sex-response cycles. J Sex Marital Ther 2001;27:33–43.
2. Berman JR, Berman LA, Toler SM, Gill J, Haughie S. Sildenafil Study Group. Safety and efficacy of sildenafil citrate for the treatment of female sexual arousal disorder: a double-blind placebo controlled study. J Urol 2003;170(6 Pt 1):2333–8.

Further reading

Dunn ME. Psychological perspectives of sex and aging. Am J Cardiol 1988; 61:24–6H.

Hakim LS, Platt, D. The Couple's Disease: Finding a Cure for Your Lost Love Life. Delary Beach, FL: DHP Publishers, 2003.

Lue TF. Erectile dysfunction. N Engl J Med 2000;342:1802–13.

McCarthy BW. Relapse prevention strategies and techniques with erectile dysfunction. J Sex Marital Ther 2001;27:1–8.

Chapter 16

Assessment of the chronic pelvic pain patient

Jonathan D Kaye, Brian A VanderBrink and
Robert M Moldwin

Introduction

Chronic pelvic pain (CPP) is a problem of significant magnitude. Up to 33% of female patients report having had CPP in their lifetime.[1] A poll of 5263 women revealed that 14.7% complained of CPP. Within this group of individuals, 11% limited their home activity due to CPP, 11.9% limited their sexual activity, and 15.8% took medication for this problem.[2] Chronic pelvic pain is the major indication for gynecologic laparoscopy in 15–40% of cases.[3]

Interpreting a patient's description of acute pain can be difficult. For the patient with chronic pelvic pain, this endeavor is yet more challenging. Misdiagnosis is common, often leading to both physician and patient frustration. A detailed history and physical examination are overwhelmingly the most important factors in achieving an accurate diagnosis. Likewise, understanding the pathophysiology and varied manifestations of chronic pain is essential in generating a complete differential diagnosis.

The varied forms of pain

The taxonomy of pain may be based upon factors as varied as pathophysiology, chronicity, site, or etiology. For the purposes of this discussion, four clinically useful classes are somatic, visceral, neuropathic, and referred pain.

Somatic pain is easily localized, well discriminated, circumscribed, and may be distributed along dermatomes. Examples of somatic pain are a cut on the finger or stub of the toe. By contrast, visceral pain is often more diffuse and may be difficult for the patient to localize. It is the most common type of pain encountered in treating patients with pelvic pain. Visceral pain is transmitted by small-diameter unmyelinated and myelinated pain fibers (C and Aδ fibers, respectively) that travel with the axons of the autonomic nervous system and project to visceral input association neurons of the brainstem. Strong contractions of the gastrointestinal system, distention, or ischemia affecting the walls of the viscera can induce severe visceral pain. Solid viscera typically have less sensitivity than hollow viscera in response to noxious stimuli. Visceral pain is typically accompanied or manifested by autonomic responses such as nausea, vomiting, sweating, and pallor. Common examples of visceral pain are renal colic, pain caused by chole-cystitis, early acute appendicitis, and ulcer pain. Referred pain, which is pain sensed in a different location than the 'pain generator,' is a common finding in those suffering visceral pain.

Neuropathic pain is produced by altered structure and/or function within the central or peripheral nervous system. Neuropathic pain is the result of an injury or malfunction in the peripheral or central nervous system.[4] Nerves can be infiltrated or compressed by tumors, strangulated by scar tis-sue, or inflamed by infection. This pain is often triggered by an injury; but this injury may or may not involve obvious damage to the nervous system. The pain frequently has burning, lancinating, or electric shock qualities. Persistent allodynia, pain resulting from a nonpainful stimulus such as a light touch, is also a common characteristic of neuropathic pain.

Neuropathic pain may persist for months or years beyond the apparent healing of any damaged tissues. In this setting, pain signals no longer repre-sent an alarm in response to ongoing or impending injury; rather, the alarm system itself is malfunctioning. An example of neuropathic pain is post-herpetic neuralgia. Other patients with neuropathic pain may have severe, spontaneous pain without allodynia, possibly secondary to increased sponta-neous activity in deafferented central neurons or reorganization of central connections. An imbalance involving loss of large inhibitory fibers and an intact or increased number of small excitatory fibers has been suggested.[5] Neuropathic pain is frequently chronic, and tends to have a less robust response to treatment with opioids, but may respond well to other drugs such as antiseizure and antidepressant medications. Usually, neuropathic problems are not fully reversible, but partial improvement is often possible with proper treatment.

A common problem that often confounds diagnosis is referral of pain. Referred pain is pain perceived at a site different from its point of origin but innervated by the same spinal segment. It is hypothesized that visceral and somatic afferent neurons converge on the same dorsal horn projection neu-rons (convergence-projection hypothesis).[6] For this reason, it can be diffi-cult for the brain to correctly identify the original source of pain. For example, a female with a ureteral stone may complain of ipsilateral labial pain. This is secondary to visceral afferent nociceptors within the ureter converging on the same pain-projection neurons as the afferents from the labia in which the pain is perceived. The brain has no way to discriminate the actual source of the input and mistakenly projects the sensation to the somatic structure[7] (Figure 16.1).

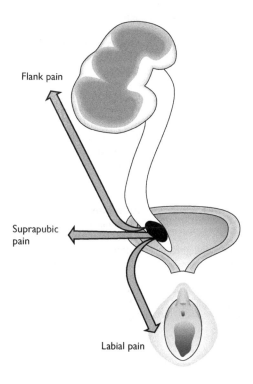

Flank pain

Suprapubic pain

Labial pain

Figure 16.1 An obstructing ureteral stone associated with pain perception at multiple sites. Courtesy of Dr R Moldwin.

Evaluation of chronic pelvic pain

As the complex pathophysiology of chronic pain suggests, accurately diagnosing the CPP patient can be extremely challenging, and is complicated further by a daunting differential diagnosis (Table 16.1). An accurate history is the single most important part of the patient's evaluation. Pertinent information regarding urologic, gynecologic, gastrointestinal, musculoskeletal, and neurologic systems must be elicited in order to initiate goal-directed therapy. The specific nature, location, and radiation of the pain, as well as its temporal relationship to any inciting event or cyclic pattern, must be noted. The social and psychological causes and effects of the pain must be explored. Ultimately, issues discussed may help guide therapy and facilitate rapport, and the discussion itself may prove therapeutic.[8]

CPP patients frequently have other systemic complaints. For reasons not entirely clear, chronic pain often encompasses a progressively larger

Table 16.1 Differential diagnoses of chronic pelvic pain in the female patient

Urologic
Bladder neoplasm
Chronic urinary tract infection
Detrusor-sphincter dyssynergia
Interstitial cystitis
Radiation cystitis
Recurrent acute cystitis
Recurrent acute urethritis
Urethral caruncle
Urethral diverticulum
Urethral syndrome
Urolithiasis

Gynecologic (extrauterine)
Adhesions
Adnexal cysts
Chlamydial endometritis or salpingitis
Chronic ectopic pregnancy
Endometriosis
Endosalpingitis
Ovarian retention syndrome
Pelvic congestion syndrome
Postoperative peritoneal cyst
Residual accessory ovary
Tuberculous salpingitis

Gynecologic (uterine)
Adenomyoma
Atypical dysmenorrhea or ovulatory pain
Cervical stenosis
Chronic endometritis
Endometrial or cervical polyps
Intrauterine contraceptive device
Genital prolapse
Leiomyomata

Gastrointestinal
Chronic intermittent bowel obstruction
Colitis
Colonic carcinoma
Constipation
Diverticular disease
Hernias
Inflammatory bowel disease
Intestinal ischemia
Irritable bowel syndrome

Musculoskeletal
Abdominal wall myofascial pain
Chronic coccygeal pain
Compression of lumbar vertebrae
Degenerative joint disease
Disk herniation
Faulty or poor posture
Fibromyositis
Lower back pain
Muscular sprains and strains
Neoplasia spinal cord or sacral nerve
Neuralgia
Pelvic floor dysfunction (levator ani spasm)
Piriformis syndrome
Rectus tendon strain
Spondylosis

Miscellaneous
Abdominal cutaneous nerve entrapment in
surgical scar
Abdominal epilepsy
Abdominal migraine
Depression
Familial Mediterranean fever
Neurologic dysfunction
Porphyria
Shingles
Sleep disturbances
Somatic referral

Reproduced with permission from Howard et al.[8]

anatomic area.[8] For example, up to 90% of CPP patients complain of back-aches and 60% endorse headaches.[9] Because of the common innervation of various urologic, gynecologic, gastrointestinal, and musculoskeletal structures, the location of a patient's pain is often misleading. Severe colonic distention typically localizes to its corresponding abdominal quadrant, but due to the length of the colonic mesentery, this pattern does not always hold.[10] Severe midline or infraumbilical pain may emanate from the uterus, adnexal structures, and lower urinary tract (Table 16.2). Small bowel pain tends to localize to the periumbilical area, whereas bladder and vaginal pain localize over the mons pubis or groin. Lower sacral and posterior midline pain can emanate from the uterosacral ligaments, posterior cul-de-sac, or cervix. Concomitant ventral and dorsal pain suggest intrapelvic pathology, whereas isolated back pain is rarely urologic, gynecologic, or gastrointestinal in origin.[12,13]

The lack of reliability of pain location is born out by Baker and Symonds' series of 60 women with CPP and negative laparoscopy: 45% had unilateral pain, 20% had bilateral pain, and 35% generalized pain.[14] However, Kresch reported 83% of his subjects to have positive laparoscopic findings, most of whom described their pain's location to be unchanged for at least 6 months.[15] Interestingly, Peters found that performing laparoscopy in women with prior history of negative laparoscopy did not improve their outcome any more than multidisciplinary pain therapy without laparoscopy.[16]

Even with the location of a patient's pain being misleading on occasion, certain salient features of the history and physical examination can assist the clinician in arriving at the correct diagnosis (Tables 16.3 and 16.4).

Table 16.2 Referred sites of pain from pelvic viscera

Structure	Segmental innervation	Potential site of referred pain
Ovaries	T10–T11	Lower abdomen, lower back
Uterus	T10–L1	Lower abdomen, lower back
Fallopian tubes	T10–L1	Lower abdomen, lower back
Perineum	S2–S4	Sacral apex, suprapubic region, rectum
External genitalia	L1–L2, S3–S4	Lower abdomen, medial anterior thigh, sacrum
Kidney	T10–L1	Ipsilateral lower back, upper abdomen
Bladder	T11–L2, S2–S4	Thoracolumbar, sacrococcygeal, suprapubic regions
Ureters	T11–L2, S2–S4	Groin, upper and lower abdomen Suprapubic, anteromedial thigh, thoracolumbar regions

Reproduced with permission from King et al.[11]

Table 16.3 Specific patient complaints regarding chronic pelvic pain and associated common diagnoses

Symptoms	Abbreviated differential diagnosis
Pain worsening premenstrually and throughout menses	Endometriosis
Pain accompanied by poor urinary flow/ urinary hesitancy and constipation	Pelvic floor or bladder neck dysfunction; anatomic obstruction, i.e. prolapsing cystocele
Dysuria, dyspareunia, urinary dribbling	Urethral diverticulum; urethritis
Pain with radiation to lower extremities	Spinal pathology (cord compression, stenosis, etc.)
Pain decreased while supine, increased while upright	Pelvic congestion syndrome, pelvic prolapse
Lateralized pain and hematuria	Urolithiasis, urinary tract obstruction, neoplasm
Crampy abdominal pain and alternating diarrhea/constipation	Irritable bowel syndrome; diverticular disease
Entry dyspareunia	Lichen sclerosis, atrophic vaginitis, vulvodynia
Deep dyspareunia	Pelvic inflammatory disease, interstitial cystitis, endometriosis, pelvic floor spasm
Increased pain with bladder filling, urinary frequency, and nocturia	Interstitial cystitis or other bladder pathology

Further diagnostic testing should be performed on the basis of suspected pathology. For example, a patient presenting with low-volume, day and nighttime urinary frequency with increased pelvic pain/discomfort with bladder filling might have interstitial cystitis. A urinalysis would be mandated in this situation to exclude other pathologies, i.e. bladder cancer, urinary tract infection, etc. The clinician should consider obtaining a urine specimen for cytologic examination in the older patient or one with a long smoking history. Further diagnostic evaluation to demonstrate the bladder as the 'pain generator' might include the use of bladder hydrodistention under anesthesia or the intravesical instillation of potassium chloride (causes an increase in pelvic pain in many interstitial cystitis patients). Another method to diagnose pain of bladder origin is the intravesical instillation of anesthetics. In this instance, a significant decrease in pain strongly suggests pain of bladder origin. Intravesical instillation of about 30 ml of a 1:1 solution of 0.5% bupivacaine and 2% lidocaine reduced pain by >50%

Table 16.4 Physical examination findings in chronic pelvic pain patients and associated common diagnoses

Signs	Abbreviated differential diagnosis
Discrete abdominal wall tenderness	Ventral hernia
Midline suprapubic tenderness	Urinary retention, interstitial cystitis, pelvic inflammatory disease
Lateralized lower quadrant tenderness	Adnexal pathology, colonic diverticular disease, urolithiasis
Introital lesions/vaginal discharge	Vaginitis, nonspecific vulvovaginitis (vulvodynia), lichen sclerosis
Anterior vaginal wall tenderness	Urethral diverticulum, urethritis, interstitial cystitis
Pelvic floor muscular tenderness associated with 'trigger points'	Pelvic floor spasm
Uterosacral ligament nodularity and pain to palpation	Endometriosis

in 77% of interstitial cystitis patients studied. The only adverse effect infrequently encountered was short-lived urinary retention.[17] A diagnosis of pelvic congestion syndrome might be entertained in the patient who has no voiding or gastroenterologic complaints, but describes her pelvic pain to worsen with sitting and standing and markedly decrease in the supine position. In this instance, pelvic ultrasonography or pelvic venography should be considered. The clinician might consider magnetic resonance imaging (MRI) of the spine in the CPP patient with no obvious pelvic pathology, but who describes lower extremity radiation of her pain.

Conclusion

Chronic pelvic pain often poses a frustrating clinical situation to both the patient and clinician. In many instances, the patient has sought advice from multiple clinicians and has been studied with enumerable and frequently fruitless diagnostic tests. Knowledge of the body's pain perception mechanisms and proficient patient interviewing skills are of paramount importance in formulating an effective plan for further management. In the event that therapy applied to a diagnosed condition fails, one must consider clinical re-evaluation.

References

1. Walker EA, Katon WJ, Jemelka R. The prevalence of chronic pelvic pain and irritable bowel syndrome in two university clinics. J Psychosom Obstet Gynecol 1991;12:65–75.
2. Mathias SD, Kuppermann M, Liberman RF, Lipschutz RC, Steege JF. Chronic pelvic pain: prevalence, health-related quality of life, and economic correlates. Obstet Gynecol 1996;87:321–7.
3. Hulka JF, Peterson HB, Phillips JM, Surrey MW. Operative laparoscopy. American Association of Gynecologic Laparoscopists 1991 membership survey. J Reprod Med 1993;38:569–71.
4. Galer BS. Neuropathic pain of peripheral origin: advances in pharmacologic treatment. Neurology 1995;45:S17–19.
5. Nurmikko T. Clinical features and pathophysiologic mechanisms of postherpetic neuralgia. Neurology 1995;45(12 Suppl 8): S54–5.
6. Wall PD, Melzack R, eds. Textbook of Pain, 3d edn. New York: Churchill Livingstone, 1994.
7. Basbaum AI, Fields HL. Endogenous pain control systems: brainstem spinal pathways and endorphin circuitry. Annu Rev Neurosci 1984;7:309–38.
8. Howard FM, Ahmed EM. Taking a history. In: Howard FM, ed. Pelvic Pain. Philadelphia: Lippincott, Williams & Wilkins, 2000.
9. Reiter RC. Chronic pelvic pain. Clin Obstet Gybecol 1990;33:117–18.
10. Rapkin AJ, Mayer EA. Gastroenterologic causes of chronic pelvic pain. Obstet Gynecol Clin North Am 1993;20:663–83.
11. King PM, Myers CA, Ling FW, Rosenthal RH. Musculoskeletal factors in chronic pelvic pain. J Psychosom Obstet Gynecol 1991;12:87.
12. Baker PK, Musculoskeletal problems. In: Steege, JF, Metzger, DA, Levy, BS, eds. Chronic Pelvic Pain. Philadelphia: WB Saunders, 1998.
13. Baker PB. Musculoskeletal origins of chronic pelvic pain. Obstet Gynecol Clin North Am 1993;20:719.
14. Baker PB, Symonds EM. The resolution of chronic pelvic pain after normal laparoscopic findings. Am J Obstet Gynecol 1992;166 835–56.
15. Kresch AJ, Seifer DB, Sachs LB, Barrese I. Laparoscopy in 100 women with chronic pelvic pain. Obstet Gynecol 1984;64:672–4.
16. Peters AA, van Dorst E, Jellis B, et al. A randomized clinical trial to compare two different approaches in women with chronic pelvic pain. Obstet Gynecol 1991;77:740–4.
17. Moldwin R, Brettschneider N. The use of intravesical anesthetics to aid in the diagnosis of interstitial cystitis. NIDDK IC Forum: Research Insights into Interstitial Cystitis: A Basic Clinical Science Symposium, 10/30–11/1/03.

Chapter 17

Complications of pelvic floor surgery

Usama Khater, Erin E Katz and Gamal Ghoniem

Introduction

Surgery is an effective treatment of pelvic floor disorders when there is an anatomic defect. Any surgical procedure can result in immediate, delayed, general, or specific complications. Some complications are specific to pelvic surgeries like obstructive symptoms after anti-incontinence procedures and injuries of the surrounding structures. The female genital and urinary tracts are closely related, so the potential for injury to one must always be considered when operating on the other. Most complications are addressed in another chapter. The following are examples of pelvic floor surgical procedures with their related complications.

Anti-incontinence procedures

Surgical intervention for the treatment of stress urinary incontinence has evolved over time. The majority of procedures performed today are minimally invasive, and can be performed as an outpatient or office procedure. Like any surgical procedure, the most common complications include subsequent infection or bleeding; however, there are a few complications that are specific to urinary incontinence surgery.

Traditionally, bulking agents have been utilized to treat patients with stress urinary incontinence secondary to intrinsic sphincter deficiency (ISD) versus patients who have urethral hypermobility. Patients with ISD experience high-grade urinary leakage with a low abdominal leak point pressure during minimal exertion.

Collagen

Contigen is a US FDA (Food and Drug Administration)-approved highly purified bovine glutaraldehyde cross-linked collagen. Intradermal skin testing 4 weeks prior to the injection is required to evaluate for a hypersensitivity reaction. The most common complication reported with collagen injection is transient urinary retention. Urinary tract infections, hematuria, and de novo urgency have also been reported. Patients with pre-existing connective tissue disorders are at an increased risk of hypersensitivity reactions, accelerated implant biodegradation, and exacerbation of their disease, thought to be due to an exacerbation of cell-mediated immunity. Development of a sterile abscess at the injection site has also been reported with collagen injections.

Teflon

Teflon is made of small particles (<100 μm) that are permanent. This material is not FDA approved in the United States due to reports of distal migration of the injected material traveling to the brain, lungs, lymph nodes, kidneys, and spleen. Granuloma formation at the injection site has also been reported.

Silicone polymers

Silicone particles are suspended in a hydrogel medium that contains larger particle sizes (>100 μm). Because of the high viscosity of the mixture, and increased viscosity upon exposure to air, higher pressures are required for injection. Because of the larger particle size, migration to distal sites should be limited. This material is still pending FDA approval in the United States.

Durasphere

Durasphere is a US FDA-approved material for the use of periurethral bulking. It is a mixture of nonabsorbable pyrolytic carbon-coated zirconium oxide beads suspended in a glucan carrier gel, with a bead size of 250–300 μm. Because of its high viscosity, a large-bore needle is required for injection, leading to a higher incidence of local edema, local discomfort, transient urgency, and transient urinary retention. An embolic phenomenon can occur if Durasphere is injected in or near the periurethral venous complex; therefore, patients with a history of right-to-left intravascular shunts should be advised not to undergo injections with Durasphere.

Autologous fat

Fat harvested from liposuction has been used as a periurethral bulking agent; however, the durability of aspirated adipocytes is poor, leading to disappointing results. Although de novo urgency and urinary tract infections have been reported, the major complication of autologous fat injection is a fat embolic event (Table 17.1).

Table 17.1 Bulking agents

Bulking agent	Trade name	Company	FDA approval
Collagen	Contigen	CR Bard	Approved
Carbon-coated zircronium oxide beads	Durasphere	Boston Scientific	Approved
Ethylene vinyl alcohol copolymer	Uryx		
	Macroplastique	Uroplasty Inc.	Pending
	Zudex		Pending

Mid-urethral slings

Minimally invasive mid-urethral slings have become the mainstay of treatment for women with stress urinary incontinence due to hypermobility and can be performed via lower abdomen or through the obturator foramen. There is no standardized method of determining proper tension of the sling, but success depends on tensionless placement of the sling. Transient obstructive urinary retention is the most common complication, and most are managed with timed voiding, double voiding, and self clean intermittent catheterization. A small percentage of patients (2.8–10%) experience prolonged urinary retention and require surgical urethrolysis and release of the sling material to restore spontaneous voiding.[1] Another complication is the development of de novo urge incontinence. Reduction of obstructive complications has been achieved by adopting the transobturator technique (TOT).

An uncommon but serious complication that has been reported in the literature is bowel perforation during insertion of a tension-free vaginal tape (TVT) (Gynecare, Ethicon, Inc., New Brunswick, NJ) and Sparc (American Medical Systems, Minnetonka, MN) trocar through the retropubic space.[2] Any patient with a prior history of abdominal or pelvic surgery is at a greater risk of this complication due to intestinal loops adherent to the pubic symphysis or in the space of Retzius. Preoperative imaging prior to the transabdominal approach may be prudent, and opting for a transobturator approach would eliminate this potential complication. Other reported complications from a transabdominal approach include iliac and femoral artery and vein injuries, hemorrhage, pelvic hematoma, obturator nerve injury, bladder perforation, bladder calculi, and erosion of the vagina, urethra, and bladder. Transobturator techniques avoid major vessels, nerves, and viscera, making it a safer procedure.

Postoperative polypropylene mesh erosion into the vagina and/or urethra has been reported. Patients usually complain of persistent vaginal discharge postoperatively; however, asymptomatic mesh erosion can be diagnosed during a routine pelvic examination. Patients may also present with vaginal or pelvic pain, vaginal bleeding, or recurrent urinary tract infections. Treatment of erosion is controversial; however, most experts would agree that urethral or bladder erosion should be managed with surgical removal of the mesh. Small vaginal erosions may be managed with surgical excision or managed conservatively with close observation, resulting in complete spontaneous healing.[3]

Traditional pubovaginal slings

Traditionally, sling procedures for stress urinary incontinence involved suspension of the bladder neck and proximal urethra, which require a more extensive dissection and inpatient hospital stay. Sling material includes autologous grafts such as rectus fascia, fascia lata, vaginal wall, round ligament and dermis, allografts, xenografts, and synthetic material. The major risk with harvesting autologous fascia has been associated with wound infection, hematoma, and entrapment of the genitofemoral nerve with the rectus fascia and the perineal nerve with the fascia lata.[4] As with the minimally invasive slings, there is a risk of transient urinary retention, de novo urge incontinence, and permanent urinary retention requiring a surgical release of the sling. If bone anchors are utilized, complications such as chronic pelvic pain, retropubic abscess, osteitis pubis, and osteomyelitis have been reported.

Allograft materials such as cadaveric fascia and cadaveric dermis have eliminated the complications associated with autologous fascia harvesting. Although remote, there is a risk of transmission of prion disease.

Retropubic colposuspension

Retropubic procedures were the mainstay of treatment of stress urinary incontinence until the minimally invasive, mid-urethral slings were introduced. These procedures include Burch colposuspension, Marshall–Marchetti–Krantz (MMK) paravaginal repair, and needle urethropexy. The main goal of these procedures was to support the bladder neck and proximal urethra in a retropubic position. Today, retropubic procedures can be done open or laparoscopically; however, laparoscopic procedures will not be discussed in this chapter.

Most retropubic procedures utilize two permanent sutures on each side of the mid-urethra and bladder neck, which are passed through Cooper's ligament and tied without tension. Intraoperatively, injury to the external iliac veins can result during placement of sutures. The most common complication with these procedures is transient urinary retention. De novo urge incontinence and worsening of existing urgency and urge incontinence, and the development of an enterocele, are also associated with retropubic colposuspensions. Patients who are obese, menopausal, or have undergone prior hysterectomy or any anti-incontinence procedure are at an increased risk of surgical failure.

Complications of pelvic floor prolapse surgery

Cystocele repair

The most common minor complications after an anterior colporrhaphy include recurrent cystocele, new-onset enterocele, transient urinary retention, de novo stress incontinence, and de novo urge incontinence. More serious complications include bladder injury during vaginal flap dissection or suture placement, ureteral obstruction secondary to suture passage, and injury or entrapment of the genital branch of the genitofemoral or ilioinguinal nerve. The development of dyspareunia is also a concern; however, it is more common with rectocele repairs.

Bladder injury should be repaired in a two-layer closure with cystoscopy performed to confirm bladder and ureteral integrity. Ureteral injury is excluded by both cystoscopy and visualization of indigo carmine-colored urine from each ureteral orifice.

Enterocele repair

Complications after an enterocele repair are uncommon: the most serious are rectal injury, small bowel injury, significant hemorrhage from suture passage through the levator muscle, ureteral injury, and vaginal evisceration.[5] Rectal and small bowel injuries may be avoided with meticulous dissection and careful insertion of the purse-string sutures. Correct identification of the yellow perirectal fat will aid in the prevention of rectal injuries, and avoidance of excessive pressure with retraction instruments will prevent retractor-type injury. Immediate recognition and repair of the rectum and small bowel is the mainstay of treatment.

Inadvertent bladder injury is usually identified with intraoperative cystoscopy, and repaired in two layers with delayed absorbable suture. Ureteral injuries are excluded by giving the patient intravenous indigo carmine and furosemide followed by cystoscopy and visualization of normal efflux of indigo carmine from the ureteral orifices. If there is no efflux, patency can be assured by placing a ureteral stent. Ureteral injury during an enterocele repair is most likely to occur with the placement of the purse-string suture. If a ureteral stent cannot be placed, the purse-string suture should be removed and the patient re-cystoscoped to assure patency.

Vaginal evisceration is a rare and life-threatening surgical emergency sometimes seen postoperatively after an enterocele repair. A literature review carried out by Virtanen et al[6] showed that the majority of eviscerations were after transabdominal repairs of the enterocele. Evisceration occurs through the vaginal cuff, and can be avoided by careful vaginal cuff closure and complete obliteration of the peritoneal sac.

Rectocele repair

Minor complications after posterior compartment surgery are persistent or worsening bowel symptoms such as constipation, incomplete evacuation, and fecal incontinence. Dyspareunia or apareunia can also occur after a rectocele repair. This is thought to be secondary to levator plication. Excessive tightness or narrowing of the introitus and vagina can also occur, contributing to dyspareunia symptoms. A more serious injury is a rectal injury. Again, immediate identification and repair of the injury with a two-layer closure using delayed absorbable suture is the treatment of choice.

Sacrospinous ligament fixation

Sacrospinous ligament fixation is used in transvaginal repair of vault prolapse. Many important structures in close proximity to the ligament must be avoided during the procedure. The pudendal vessels and nerve and the nerve to the obturator internus all travel around the ischial spine. The hypogastric vessels, sciatic nerve, and gluteal artery are in close proximity to the sacrospinous ligament.

Minor complications include recurrent pelvic relaxation, such as anterior and posterior vaginal wall prolapses. Genital pain or discomfort most commonly result from small nerve entrapment, and the complication is usually transient. Vaginal narrowing, leading to sexual dysfunction, can also occur. More serious injuries are hemorrhage that requires transfusion and bladder and rectal injuries that require immediate repair. Spontaneous resolution of chronic gluteal pain, or pudendal, sciatic, or lumbar plexus neuropathies can also occur.

Bladder substitution and augmentation

Bladder carcinoma is the second most common genitourinary tumor, and in the United States nearly 55 000 patients are diagnosed annually, with 12 000 dying from the disease.[7] Radical cystectomy with urinary diversion is the standard treatment of invasive bladder cancer.

Ileal Conduit (IC)

Ileal conduit (IC) urinary diversion, which is technically the simplest type of diversion, is associated with the least amount of postoperative complications. It is a noncontinent cutaneous diversion that requires an external urinary collecting device. An isolated 15 cm segment of ileum 15 cm distal to the ileocecal valve, is used. The distal end of the conduit is secured to the anterior abdominal wall as a stoma, along with direct mucosal-to-mucosal ureteroenteric anastomosis to the proximal end of the conduit. Most complications are related to the stoma, and the majority of these can be avoided by careful preoperative selection and marking of the stoma site. An ill-fitting external collection device, resulting from a stoma placed in a skin crease, belt line, or over pre-existing scars, can lead to persistent urinary leakage, skin breakdown, and dermatitis. A poorly fitted device leads to chronic skin exposure to alkaline urine, causing irritation and blistering. Patient neglect of the stoma, poor hygiene, and the inability to properly care for the stoma site may contribute to chronic skin problems.

Other complications related to the stoma include parastomal hernias, stomal stenosis, and retraction of the stoma. Patients are instructed to avoid straining and heavy lifting in the first 3 months after surgery, which will help prevent parastomal hernia and prolapse formation.

Continent cutaneous diversion

The Indiana pouch (IP) is a viable option for patients who have good manual dexterity, are motivated and do not want an external drainage device,

Table 17.2 Summary of the electrolyte abnormalities specific to the segment of bowel used

Intestinal segment utilized	Electrolyte abnormality	Preferred treatment
Stomach	Hypochloremic Hypokalemic Metabolic alkalosis	H_2 blockers Proton pump inhibitors
Jejunum	Hyponatremic Hyperkalemic Hypochloremic Metabolic acidosis	NaCl NaHCO$_3$
Ileum/colon	Hyperchloremic Metabolic acidosis	NaHCO$_3$ Bicitra/polycitra

but their urethra is unable to be utilized for reconstruction. The IP allows patient to remain dry for at least 4 hours without having to catheterize the stoma, and many patients can remain continent during the normal sleep interval without requiring catheterization.

The right colon and 8–10 cm of the terminal ilium is mobilized, and the terminal ileal segment is plicated to create the efferent limb for catheterization. Direct mucosal-to-mucosal ureteroenteric anastomosis in the afferent limb are performed. Early minor complications (<3 months postoperatively) that can occur with continent cutaneous diversions include dehydration, electrolyte abnormalities, superficial wound infections, prolonged ileus, hydronephrosis, pyelonephrosis, and pelvic fluid collections. Superficial wound infections may be increased in patients who undergo IP as a result of the higher bacterial count in the colon despite adequate bowel preparation prior to surgery. Late complications (>3 months postoperatively) unique to the continent cutaneous diversion include difficulty in catheterizing the stoma, intermittent urinary leakage, pouchitis, and stone formation in the pouch. Major late complications include IP to vagina fistula and ureteral stricture formation.[8]

The majority of patients who have initial difficulty catheterizing the pouch do not require surgical revision, and the difficulty resolves over time. The plicated ileal limb provides compression and urinary continence based on a competent ileocecal valve.

Urinary calculi in reservoirs have been reported to be a frequent late complication. The majority of stones can be successfully managed percutaneously. It has been found that the majority of these stones are not associated with foreign material, but due to noncompliance with clean intermittent catheterization.[9] Most of the stones contain struvite, indicating an infectious etiology. Pouch irrigation on a regular basis can minimize infection and stone formation. Surgical revision of the efferent limb is required when there is significant limb elongation due to stomal stenosis, leading to residual urine, recurrent pouch calculi, and recurrent pouchitis.

Orthotopic neobladder continent diversion

With better understanding of female pelvic anatomy and the sphincteric mechanism, lower urinary tract reconstruction with direct anastomosis to the urethra in women is a viable option. Sparing the rhabdosphincter mechanism (distal two-thirds of the female urethra) allows the patient to resume volitional voiding by Valsalva. In the postoperative period, voiding education is of paramount importance, including instruction on pelvic floor relaxation, timed voiding, and frequent follow-up visits. Traditionally, 48–60 cm of ileum, 15 cm distal to the ileocecal valve, is utilized for pouch formation, with direct anastomosis of the pouch to the native urethra, along with direct mucosal-to-mucosal ureteroenteric anastomosis.

Early minor complications that occur with orthotopic neobladders (ONBs) are similar to continent cutaneous diversions, including prolonged ileus, dehydration, electrolyte abnormalities, superficial wound infection, urinoma, and pelvic fluid collections. The most common late complications are urinary retention that requires clean intermittent catheterization, mild stress incontinence, bladder neck contracture, ONB to vagina fistula, ONB to small-bowel fistula, small-bowel obstruction, and ureteral strictures. Hautmann et al[10] described 11-year results of 363 patients following cystectomy and ileal neobladder. Early and late neobladder-related complications occurred in 15.4% and 23.4% of patients, respectively. The reoperation rate for neobladder-related complications was 0.3% (early) and 4.4% (late).

Preservation of the anterior vaginal wall, endopelvic fascia, and pubourethral ligaments should be performed, as these structures may play an important role in urinary continence and sexual function. Preservation of these structures maintains vaginal length and support, preventing pelvic descent. Placement of an omental flap may decrease fistula formation and provide additional urethral support. Anterior vaginal wall prolapse resulting in a 'pouchocele' effect with associated urinary retention has been reported.[11]

In a recent review by Fujisawa et al,[12] 11 women underwent a modified sigmoid neobladder. Their voiding pattern and continence status were evaluated at 3 months, with measured neocystourethral angles. Leaving the anterior vaginal wall intact allowed preservation of a wide neocystourethral angle (range 110–180°), thus avoiding development of a severe angle and 'hypercontinence'. It has been suggested that urinary retention may be due to the combination of a severe neocystourethral angle, a downward migration of the neobladder, and a low pressure reservoir.[13]

Urinary fistulas tend to occur early in the postoperative course. A well-vascularized omental pedicle graft interposed between the reconstructed neobladder and the vagina along with avoiding overlapping suture lines aids in the prevention of fistula formation and postoperative prolapse.

Urinary leak at the anastomotic site is greatly reduced by the use of soft Silastic ureteral stents at the time of surgery. A urinary leak may lead to periureteral fibrosis and subsequent stricture formation, leading to hydronephrosis, pyelonephritis, and/or deterioration of kidney function.[14] A left ureteral stricture formation is more common because the left ureter is tunneled under the mesentery beneath the inferior mesenteric artery, also causing slight angulation of the ureter.

Certain electrolyte abnormalities are specific to the type of bowel segment utilized. Other metabolic disturbances after a diversion include abnormal drug metabolism, altered hepatic metabolism, osteomalacia, and growth retardation. Jejunum should not be used in reconstruction to minimize these complications.

Augmentation cystoplasty

Augmentation cystoplasty can be performed in patients who suffer from severe detrusor instability combined with intractable urge incontinence, and a small bladder capacity, refractory to conservative therapy. Patients must have good manual dexterity, and be taught self-clean intermittent catheterization preoperatively. The most common enterocystoplasty is the utilization of a detubularized ileal segment anastomosed to a widely bivalved bladder; however, large-bowel cystoplasties are also performed. Minor complications include symptomatic urinary tract infections, mucus retention, prolonged ileus, chronic diarrhea, and bladder calculi. Major complications include bowel obstruction, patch necrosis, perforation of augmented bladder, malignant transformation, and metabolic disturbances.[15]

Pregnancy and augmentation

Pregnancy in patients with complex genitourinary reconstruction is becoming more common. Women with a history of congenital anomalies and neurogenic bladder who have undergone augmentation cystoplasty at a young age are now reaching potential childbearing age. Little work has been done to study bladder function during the course of pregnancy. The most common complication in these patients during pregnancy is a urinary tract infection. Important risk factors include increased residual urine, ureteral dilatation, and diminished tone of the upper tract. Any cases of a urinary tract infection must be treated promptly to prevent premature labor and fetal morbidity. Renal function must be monitored closely, including serial serum creatinine and uric acid levels to detect pre-eclampsia.

Some urologists recommend a cesarean section for delivery to avoid disruption of the continence mechanism during a vaginal delivery.[16–18] This is especially true if a patient has undergone extensive bladder neck repair. However, multiple studies have shown successful pregnancies with spontaneous vaginal deliveries with no detrimental effect on all types of urinary diversions. A study by Schilling et al showed that the mesenteric pedicle for diversions extended cranially and laterally away from the uterus, and the pedicle of augmented bladders tended to cover the uterus.[19] Interestingly, neither diversion type prevented the rise of the uterus during pregnancy. It is speculated that a gradual increase in the size of the uterus during pregnancy allows the mesentery to stretch slowly, accommodating the uterus. A study by Quennevilk et al reported three cases of women who had an ileocystoplasty combined with a modified fascial sling, delivered vaginally, and continence was unchanged.[20]

If a cesarean section is indicated, it should be done electively, and a urologist with knowledge of the anatomy of the cystoplasty should be present. The mesenteric blood supply to the cystoplasty must be avoided. The mesentery of the augmented bladder may be pushed aside by the uterus, or it may be draped over it. The mesenteric blood supply can be interrupted during the procedure and may not be obvious at the time of surgery or immediately afterward. Revision of the enterocystoplasty might be needed if the enteric segment contracts and the bladder capacity is reduced.

Pregnancy and vaginal delivery after augmentation cystoplasty, incontinent diversions, and continent diversions is possible. Urologists and obstetricians should be aware of the potential complications of pregnancy and delivery.

Complications related to patient positioning

The majority of anti-incontinence surgeries are performed with the patient in a dorsal lithotomy position. Patients in an improper dorsal lithotomy and Trendelenburg position for longer than 4 hours are at an increased risk of neuropraxia, deep vein thrombosis, and compartment syndrome.[21] A combination of a head-down position, angulation of the hips and lower limbs, with bad calf supports decreases arterial perfusion and increases intracompartmental pressure, increasing the risk of significant complications. Ideally, the patient should be positioned by the surgeon, utilizing Allen stirrups, and assuring no leg overflexion. If the anticipated procedure takes longer than 4 hours, the legs should be removed from the stirrups every 2 hours to prevent reperfusion injury.

Sequelae from nerve injury include foot drop, paresthesia, ankle equines, and claw or hammer toes, all of which lead to gait impairment. Other risk factors for the development of nerve damage include patients with narrow pelvis, thin patients, extensive retroperitoneal pelvic dissection, Pfannenstiel incision beyond the edge of the rectus muscle, and the use of shoulder braces. Nerve damage from improper retractor placement can also occur. Ileoinguinal nerve entrapment can result from suture placement. Patients will experience pain and difficulty in walking but can be treated by excision of the offending suture.[22]

Prevention

Good surgical training, thorough preoperative history and diagnostic work-up, in addition to the awareness of the anatomy of pelvis, are the best ways to avoid complications.

References

1. Leach GE, Dmochowski RR, Appell RA, et al. Female Stress Urinary Incontinence Clinical Guidelines Panel summary report on surgical management of female stress urinary incontinence. The American Urological Association. J Urol 1997;158:875–80.
2. Leboeuf L, Tellez C, Ead D, Gousse A. Complication of bowel perforation during insertion of tension-free vaginal tape. J Urol. 2003;170(4):1310–1.
3. Kobashi K, Govier F. Management of vaginal erosion of polypropylene mesh slings. J Urol. 2003;169(6):2242–3.
4. Manoj M. Ghoniem GM. Ilioinguinal nerve entrapment following needle bladder suspension procedures. Urology 1994;44(3):447–50.
5. Kobashi KC, Leach GE. Pelvic prolapse. J Urol 2000;164(6):1879–90.
6. Virtanen HS, Ekholm E, Kiilholma PJ. Evisceration after enterocele repair: a rare complication of vaginal surgery. Urogynecol J Pelvic Floor Dysfunct 1996; 7:344–7.
7. Landis SH, Murray T, Bolden S, Wingo PA. Cancer statistics, 1999. CA Cancer J Clin 1999;49(1):8–31.
8. Lampel A, Thuroff J. Urologic intestinal reservoirs: the continent outlet. Curr Conc Urol 1998;8(3):221.
9. Terai A, Ueda T, Kakehi Y, et al. Urinary calculi as a late complication of the Indiana continent urinary diversion: comparison with the Koch pouch procedure. J Urol 1996;155(1):66–8.
10. Hautmann RE, de Petriconi R, Gottfried HW, et al. The ileal neobladder: complications and functional results in 363 patients after 11 years of followup. J Urol 1999;161(2):427–8.
11. Stenzl A, Colleselli K, Poisel S, et al. Rationale and technique of nerve sparing radical cystectomy before an orthotopic neobladder in women. J Urol 1995;154(6):2044–9.
12. Fujisawa M, Gotoh A, Miyazaki S, et al. Sigmoid neobladder in women after radical cystectomy. J Urol 2000;163(5):1505–9.
13. Ali-El-dein B, Gomha M, Ghoniem M. Critical evaluation of the problem of chronic urinary retention after orthotopic bladder substitution in women. J Urol 2002;168(2):587–92.
14. Stampfer DS, McDougal WS, McGovern FJ. The use of in bowel urology. Metabolic and nutritional complications. Urol Clin North Am 1997; 24(4):715–22.
15. Quek M, Ginsberg D. Long-term urodynamics followup of bladder augmentation for neurogenic bladder. J Urol 2003;169(1):195–8.
16. Hill DE, Kramer SA. Management of pregnancy after augmentation cystoplasty. J Urol 1990;144:457–9.
17. Fenn N, Barrington JW, Stephenson TP. Clam enterocystoplasty and pregnancy. Br J Urol 1995;75:85–6.
18. Kennedy WA 2nd, Hensle TW, Reiley EA, Fox HE, Haus T. Pregnancy after orthotopic continent urinary diversion. Surg Gynecol Obstet 1993;177:405–9.
19. Schilling A, Krawczak G, Friesen A, Kruse H. Pregnancy in a patient with an ileal substitute bladder followed by severe destabilization of the pelvic support. J Urol 1996;155:1389–90.

20. Quenneville V, Beurton D, Thomas L, Fontaine E. Pregnancy and vaginal delivery after augmentation cystoplasty. Br J Urol 2003;91:893–4.
21. Raza A, Byrne D, Townell N. Lower limb (well leg) compartment syndrome after urological pelvic surgery. J Urol. 2004;171(1):5–11.
22. Monga M, Ghoniem GM. Ilioinguinal nerve entrapment following needle bladder suspension procedures. Urology 1994;44(3):447–50.

Chapter 18

Interstitial cystitis

Gamal Ghoniem and Usama Khater

Introduction

Interstitial cystitis (IC) is a chronic, debilitating disease of the urinary bladder characterized by urinary frequency, nocturia, urgency, and frequently pain. It affects more females than males by a ratio of approximately 10:1.[1] Recently, the International Continence Society (ICS) has developed a somewhat broader term for IC, described as 'IC-painful bladder syndrome'. This new term is defined as the complaint of suprapubic pain related to bladder filling, and is accompanied by other symptoms, such as increased daytime and night-time frequency in the absence of proven urinary infection or other obvious pathology.[2] The true prevalence of IC is not determined and it may be underestimated. In 1997, Jones and Nyberg estimated that up to 1 million patients in the United States suffer from IC, and many of them are unable to cope with day-to-day activities.[3]

Etiology and pathogenesis

Despite aggressive investigation in the past two decades, the cause and pathophysiology of the disease remain elusive. Several theories of its pathogenesis have been proposed, but none fully account for the manifestation of the disease.

Occult infection

Attempts to show an infectious etiology go back to the dawn of the disease, but the case has never been a strong one. Bacterial, viral, and fungal studies were performed on IC patients, and they failed to substantiate an infectious etiology. Infection with 'atypical' or fastidious organisms has been proposed by numerous investigators. Domingue and Ghoniem suggested that even if the organisms are not causative agents, their presence may lead to immune and host cell responses that could initiate or exacerbate an inflammatory state.[4]

Defective mucosal layer (epithelial dysfunction)

The healthy bladder surface is coated by a thin mucinous substance, termed bladder surface mucin (BSM), which is composed of numerous sulfonated glycosaminoglycans (GAGs) and glycoprotein. This mucus lining prevents urine and its contents from leaking through the urothelium and damaging the underlying nerves and muscles. In IC patients, this layer is defective and the epithelium is abnormally permeable. As a result, potentially toxic substances in urine are permitted to permeate the bladder muscle, depolarizing sensory nerves and causing the symptoms of IC. One of the urine constituents is potassium (K^+), which is highly toxic to the bladder muscularis. Therefore, a potassium sensitivity test has been developed to diagnose IC.

Mast cell involvement

Simmons, in 1961, was the first to suggest mast cells as a cause of IC.[5] Mast cells contain cytoplasmic granules, which in turn contain substances such as histamine, leukotrienes, prostaglandins, and tryptases. All these substances are capable of stimulating inflammation. Mastocytosis has been reported in the bladders of 30–65% of patients with IC.[6,7] Elevated levels of histamine and its metabolites in the urine of IC patients were reported by some investigators. Others found overlap or no difference in urinary histamine excretions in IC patients and controls.[8,9] Whether mast cells have a primary or secondary role in the etiology of IC is not exactly known.

Neurogenic mechanism

Neurogenic inflammation is a process by which nerves may secrete inflammatory mediators, resulting in local inflammation and/or hyperalgesia. This pathogenesis is described in IC as well as in other painful syndromes. One central component of this mechanism is substance P, a short-chain peptide that functions as a nociceptive neurotransmitter in the central and peripheral nervous system and as an inflammatory mediator. When released by peripheral nerves (C fibers or fibers associated with pain transmission), an inflammatory cascade occurs that results in processes such as mast cell degranulation and activation of nearby nerves. Supporting the role of neurogenic inflammation in IC is the finding of increased numbers of substance P-containing nerve fibers in the bladders of IC patients.[10]

Autoimmunity and inflammation

The exact role of autoimmunity in IC remains controversial, with no clear indication of a primary role for autoimmunity as the cause of IC. Urothelial activation in IC may result in aberrant immune responses and immune activation within the bladder wall that could relate to the pathogenesis of the disease. Numerous inflammatory mediators have been studied with regard to their relation to IC. Bladder inflammation is categorized by elevated urinary interleukin-6 and activation of the kallikrein–kinin system.[11] Abdel-Mageed and Ghoniem were the first researchers to find activated nuclear factor kappa B in the bladder biopsies of IC patients.[12] This nuclear factor was also found in other inflammatory diseases such as rheumatoid arthritis, inflammatory bowel disease, and bronchial asthma. Activation of this nuclear factor was found to be responsible for the production of proinflammatory cytokines.[13]

Toxic substances in urine

The idea that the urine of IC patients carries a pathologic substance accounting for the disorder has been suggested. The initial observation that the urine of IC patients may contain pathological substances was suggested when it was found that it inhibits the proliferation of cultured human transitional cells. Keay et al determined that the urine of IC patients, specifically, contains a low-molecular-weight protein factor, an antiproliferative factor (APF), that inhibits bladder epithelium proliferation.[14]

Clinical picture

Patients can present with many symptoms. At the early stage of symptoms, they may be misdiagnosed with recurrent or chronic urinary tract infection before diagnosis of IC. These symptoms include urgency, frequency, pelvic pain, pelvic pressure, bladder spasm, dyspareunia, dysuria, awakening at night with pain, and pain that persists for many days after intercourse. The location of pain includes the vaginal area, the lower abdomen, suprapubic area, groin, or low back. Many symptoms are aggravated by menstruation and most of the patients feel that sexual intercourse exacerbates their symptoms. Pain worsens if the bladder is full and it improves with voiding. Bladder pain of IC is experienced suprapubically, in the perineum, vulva, vagina, or in the back or medial thigh.

Most patients will also have nocturia, at least 1–2 times per night.

Symptoms scores

In 1997 O'Leary et al developed a questionnaire specifically to assess IC patients.[15] The questionnaire is composed of two sections, including symptoms and problem indices. The maximum scores are 20 and 16, respectively. A second questionnaire, the University of Wisconsin IC Scale (UW-ICS), includes 7 points, with a 0 (not at all) to 6 (a lot) rating scale. The summated scale ranges from 0 to 42.[16] These questionnaires are designed to evaluate the severity of IC symptoms and their regression or progression with and without treatment.

Voiding diary

The number of daily voidings and average volume can be determined from a voiding dairy, whereas each voiding is recorded and measured by the patient (Appendix I). IC patients void an average of 16 times per day. A voiding diary can be used to document frequency and to evaluate treatment.

Diagnosis

The diagnosis of IC is suspected by the clinician after exclusion of other diseases that have a similar clinical picture, as no objective test exists. In August 1987, the National Institute of Diabetes and Digestive and Kidney Diseases (NIDDKD) established criteria to diagnose IC for research purposes.[17] Clinical application of these criteria in routine clinical practice will miss 60% of patients with IC.[18] Recently, there has been an attempt to introduce determination of the urinary marker APF into the diagnosis of IC.

Physical examination

The main goal of examination is to exclude identifiable causes that may be responsible for the patient's symptoms. Abdominal examination is usually normal in IC patients, except for occasional suprapubic tenderness. On pelvic examination, identifiable diseases can be recognized or excluded. A rectal examination should assess for other sources of perineal pain, such as anal fissure, and the presence of masses. Rectovaginal and bimanual examinations may reveal masses or implants suggestive of endometriosis. In the classic IC patient, palpation of the anterior wall reveals a tender bladder base; pelvic floor muscle spasm and tenderness are also usually found. Occasionally, trigger points may be found along the levator ani muscles.

Urinalysis and cultures are required. Urine cytology should also be obtained to rule out the possibility of carcinoma. If hematuria is found, a full urinary tract work-up should be performed to exclude malignancy.

Cystoscopy

Cystoscopy is performed to exclude other bladder pathology, including carcinoma in situ and other malignancy. In the office, cystoscopy under local anesthesia is usually normal in IC. However, cystoscopy and hydrodistention under anesthesia have more of a therapeutic than diagnostic role, as the presence of glomerulations is not specific and their absence does not exclude the diagnosis of IC. Water is infused at pressure of $80 cmH_2O$

into the bladder until filling stops. Diminished bladder capacity under anesthesia can be seen in patients with advanced forms of IC. The bladder is distended for 2–5 minutes before all irrigant is released from the bladder. Terminal bloody efflux of irrigant suggests the diagnosis of IC. The bladder is then re-examined cystoscopically. The appearance of glomerulation (petechiae) (Figure 18.1) and/or Hunner's ulcers (Figure 18.2), which appear as fissures or cracks in the epithelium, are consistent with IC. The appearance of Hunner's ulcers is not common in IC (11%), although it has been suggested that its presence is a more specific sign than glomerulation.[19] Hydrodistention has a therapeutic role, as it can relieve the IC symptoms in 30–50% of patients.[20] Normalization of urine growth factor abnormalities and APF was seen after hydrodistention.[21]

Urodynamics

Urodynamic studies are not routinely indicated in evaluation of IC patients. It can be performed if the patient's symptoms include incontinence, severe urgency, or obstructive voiding complaints. Compliance may be normal or decreased in IC patients. IC patients report pain on filling and show decreased capacity.

Potassium sensitivity test

The potassium (KCl) sensitivity test is based on the assertion that bladder epithelium is leaky in IC patients. Potassium in the urine crosses the urothelium to the submucosa and muscle layer, causing sensory nerve irritation

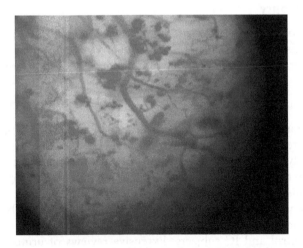

Figure 18.1 Cystoscopy following hydrodistention of the bladder, showing diffuse glomerulation. (See also color image on p. xxxii)

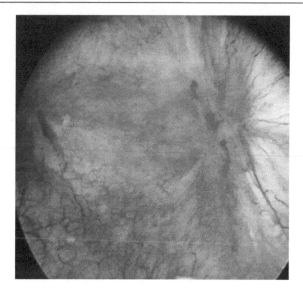

Figure 18.2 Hunner's ulcer. (See also color image on p. xxxii)

and inflammation. The IC Committee in 2003 did not recommend the KCl test because neither high sensitivity nor specificity has been established.[2]

Bladder biopsy

Bladder biopsy is not diagnostic for IC, but it is indicated to exclude other possible diseases, particularly carcinoma. Biopsy is taken during cystoscopy, after hydrodistention, to avoid bladder perforation or rupture.

Urinary markers

Many urinary substances have been described as increased or decreased in IC compared with controls. These substances, including histamine, interleukins, glycosaminoglycans, hyaluronic acid, epithelial growth factors, nerve growth factor, and others, were selected based on theorized etiologies for IC. One of the major problems of using many of these substances as diagnostic markers is that, while the levels may be statistically significantly higher or lower in IC, most of the individual values significantly overlap among control and IC subjects. Extensive reviews of urine markers have been published.[22] Glycoprotein 51 and APF did not show overlap between controls and IC patients who met NIDDKD criteria. The level of APF is detected with an indirect assay based on inhibition of H-thymidine incorporation. The sensitivity and specificity of APF were 94% and 95%, respectively.[23] APF is more likely to be a diagnostic marker for IC.

Treatment

Management of IC patients should include different approaches, as often these patients have comorbidities such as depressed mood.

Dietary modification

Avoidance of certain foods and beverages appears to improve the symptoms in many IC patients. Fluid restriction, although it will decrease the frequency, is not advised, as pain often worsens due to a higher concentration of offending agents in the urine. Urine alkalinization may help.

Oral therapy

Oral medications are used to enhance the GAG layer (pentosan polysulfate), stabilize mast cells in the bladder wall (hydroxyzine), modulate neural input (amitriptyline, gabapentin), control pain (narcotics), control inflammation (anti-inflammatory drugs), improve frequency (anticholinergics), control dysuria (phenazopyridine), and to improve sleep (zolpidem). Amitriptyline showed significant improvement in IC symptoms when compared to placebo.[24]

Intravesical therapy

Intravesical therapy can be used alone or in combination with oral therapy. Its advantages include high local drug concentration in the bladder, minimal systemic absorption, and a lack of significant systemic side-effects.

Intravesical dimethyl sulfoxide

The beneficial effect of dimethyl sulfoxide (DMSO) appears to be its ability to release and ultimately deplete substance P from the bladder wall. Initially, DMSO may exacerbate the symptoms as it may stimulate mast cell degranulation and stimulate bladder efferent pathways to cause nitric oxide release. DMSO is administered as a 50% solution or as a DMSO cocktail.[25] The solution consists of 50 ml of 50% DMSO (Rimso-50), 10 ml of sodium bicarbonate, steroid (40 mg triamcinolone), 10 000 units of heparin sulfate, and 80 mg of gentamicin. The mixture is administered and the patient is asked to hold it for 30–60 minutes. Patients may experience an initial flare-up of symptoms as a result of an increased substance P. These symptoms usually improve after 2 weeks of treatment. Therapy is ultimately discontinued when symptoms have been reduced and stabilized.

Intravesical heparin

Intravesical heparin is thought to enhance the protective feature of BSM. Heparin also has anti-inflammatory properties, inhibiting angiogenesis and proliferation of fibroblasts and smooth muscle fibers. Self-instilled 20 000 IU of heparin can be used, and no changes in coagulation studies can occur.[26] The solution is held for 30–45 minutes, and then voided. Four to 12 months is often needed to attain a beneficial response.

Anesthetic cocktail

As the bladder is suspected to be the source of pain in the IC patient, direct treatment of its surface may produce improvement of symptoms. The solution consists of bupivacaine and lidocaine. The patient is instructed to hold the solution for 30 minutes, and the instillation is repeated on a weekly basis for 8–12 weeks.

Silver nitrate and Clorpactin WCS-90

Instillation of caustic agents, including silver nitrate and oxychlorosene, is used in the treatment of IC. Success rates may vary from 50% to 80%.[27] As these agents are caustic, avoiding cystogram should be performed to exclude any vesicoureteral reflux and to avoid upper urinary tract damage. Bladder biopsy is contraindicated along with instillation of these agents to avoid perivesical extravasations.

Bacillus Calmette-Guérin

Bacillus Calmette-Guérin (BCG) is an attenuated strain of *Mycobacterium bovis*. BCG can provide a 60% improvement rate compared with 27% using a placebo.[28]

Sodium hyaluronate

Sodium hyaluronate is a highly purified salt of hyaluronic acid. Hyaluronic acid is a glycosaminoglycan component of BSM. Intravesical administration of hyaluronic acid may improve the bladder lining and further protect the bladder wall from the irritating effect of urine. It is available commercially in Europe and Canada and although under investigation in the United States, the results were inconclusive.

Capsaicin and resiniferatoxin

Capsaicin is the pungent component of capsicum, the hot pepper. Chronic application is known to be associated with C-fiber (unmyelinated nerve fibers known for transmitting painful stimuli) desensitization.

Surgical intervention

Hydrodistention

As previously mentioned, hydrodistention has therapeutic and diagnostic roles in IC. Hydrodistention may offer relief of symptoms in 30–50% of patients. The symptoms may worsen 2–3 weeks after the procedure and improve after that period. Patients with small bladder capacity under anesthesia tend to have a better response to hydrodistention than those with large capacity. The mean duration of improvement is about 3 months, while with repeating hydrodistension, the improvement may progressively decrease.[29]

Neuromodulation

Neuromodulation is a unilateral sacral nerve (S3) stimulation device (InterStim device, Medtronic, Inc., Minneapolis, MN). Neuromodulation has been approved by the FDA for treatment of urge incontinence, urinary retention, idiopathic urgency-frequency syndrome, and recently for IC.[30]

Laser resection of ulcers

Laser procedures are reserved for those patients suffering from gross inflammatory lesions of the bladder wall (Hunner's patches). In this procedure, the Nd:YAG (2neodymium: yttrium–aluminium–garnet) laser has been used for ablation of Hunner's patch ablation.

Cystectomy and urinary diversion

Cystectomy with urinary diversion is the last resort procedure, reserved for patients who have failed all other modalities of treatment and for those with small anesthetic bladder capacity. Pain may be persistent in some patients after this aggressive therapeutic approach, and before surgery is considered, patients are evaluated by the pain clinic to localize the pain. If there is evidence of central up-regulation of pain, surgery will not be performed, since it will not relieve the pain.

References

1. Hanno PM, Levin RM, Monson FC, et al. Diagnosis of interstitial cystitis [see comments]. J Urol 1990;143:278–81.
2. Allen P. Committee moves closer to revised definition of IC. Urol Times 2004;32:1–11.
3. Jones CA, Nyberg L. Epidemiology of interstitial cystitis. Urology 1997; 49:2–9.
4. Domingue GJ, Ghoniem GM. Occult infection in interstitial cystitis. In: Sant GR, ed. Interstitial cystitis. Philadelphia: Lippincott-Raven, 1997: 77–86.
5. Simmons JL. Interstitial cystitis: an explanation for the beneficial effect of an antihistamine. J Urol 1961;85:149–55.
6. Feltis JT, Perez-Marrero R, Emerson LE. Increased mast cells of bladder in suspected cases of interstitial cystitis: possible disease marker. J Urol 1987; 138:746–52.
7. Lynes WL, Flynn SD, Shortliffe LD, et al. Mast cell involvement in intestitial cystitis. J Urol 1987;138:746–52.
8. El Mansoury M, Boucher W, Sant GR, et al. Increased urine histamine and methylhistamine in interstitial cystitis. J Urol 1994;152:350–3.
9. Erickson D, Xie S, Bhavanadan VP, et al. A comparison of multiple urine markers for interstitial cystitis. J Urol 2002;167(6):2461–9.
10. Hoenfeller M, Nunues L, Schmidt RA, et al. Interstitial cystitis: increased sympathetic innervation and related neuropeptide synthesis. J Urol 1992; 147:587–91.
11. Lotz M, Villiger P, Hugli T, et al. Interleukin-6 and interstitial cystitis. J Urol 1994;152:869–73.
12. Abdel-Mageed A, Ghoniem G. Potential role of Rel/nuclear factor-kappa B in the pathogenesis of interstitial cystitis. J Urol 1998;160:2000–3.
13. Abdel-Mageed AB, Bajwa A, Shenassa BB, Human L, Ghoniem GM. NF-kappa B-dependent gene expression of proinflammatory cytokines in T24 cells: possible role in interstitial cystitis. Urol Res 2003;31:300–5.
14. Keay S, Zhang CO, Trifillis AL, et al. Decreased H-thymidine incorporation by human bladder epithelial cells following exposure to urine from interstitial cystitis patients. J Urol 1996;156:2073–8.
15. O'Leary MP, Sant GR, Fowler F, et al. The interstitial cystitis symptom index and problem index. Urology 1997;49:58–63.
16. Goin JF, Olaleye D, Peter KM, et al. Psychometeric analysis of the University of Wisconsin Interstitial Cystitis Scale: implications for use in randomized clinical trials. J Urol 1998;159:1085–90.
17. Gillenwater JY, Wein AJ. Summary of the National Institute of Arthritis, Diabetes, Digestive and Kidney Diseases Workshop on Interstitial Cystitis, National Institutes of Health, Bethesda, Maryland, August 28–29, 1987. J Urol 1988;140:203–6.
18. Hanno PM, Landis JR, Matthews-Cook Y, et al. The diagnosis of interstitial cystitis revisited: lessons learned from the National Institutes of Health Interstitial Cystitis Database study. J Urol 1999;161:553–7.
19. Messing E, Pauk D, Schaeffer A, et al. Associations among cystoscopic findings

and symptoms and physical examination findings in women enrolled in the Interstitial Cystitis Data Base (ICDB) Study. Urology 1997;49(Suppl 5A):81–5.

20. Hanno PM, Buehler J, Wein AJ. Conservative treatment of interstitial cystitis. Semin Urol 1991;9:143–7.

21. Chi TX, Zhang CO, Shoenfelt JL, et al. Bladder stretch alters urinary heparin-binding epidermal growth factor and antiproliferative factor in patients with interstitial cystitis. J Urol 2000;163:1440–4.

22. Erickson DR. Urine markers in interstitial cystitis. Urology 2001;57:15–21.

23. Keay SK, Zhang C, Shoenfelt J, et al. Sensitivity and specificity of antiproliferative factor, heparin-binding epidermal growth factor-like growth factor and epidermal growth factor as urine markers for interstitial cystitis. Urology 2001;57(6 Suppl 1):9–14.

24. van Ophoven A, Pokupic S, Heinecke A, Hertle L. A prospective, randomized, placebo controlled, double-blind study of amitriptyline for the treatment of interstitial cystitis. [Clinical Trial. Journal Article – Randomized Controlled Trial]. Journal of Urology 2004;172(2):533–6.

25. Ghoniem G, McBride D, Sood OP, et al. Clinical experience with multiagent intravesical therapy in interstitial cystitis patients unresponsive to single-agent therapy. World J Urol 1993;11:178–82.

26. Parsons CL, Housley T, Schmidt JD, et al. Treatment of interstitial cystitis with intravesical heparin. Br J Urol 1994;73:504–7.

27. Moldwin RM, Sant GR. Interstitial cystitis: a pathophysiology and treatment update. Clinical Obstet Gynecol 2002;45(1):259–72.

28. Peters KM, Diokno AC, Steinert BW, et al. The efficacy of intravesical bacillus Calmette-Guerin in the treatment of interstitial cystitis: long term follow up. J Urol 1998;159:1483–7.

29. Rofeim O, Shupp-Byrne D, Mulholand SG, et al. Increased production of bladder surface mucin due to bladder trauma. J Urol 2000;163:40.

30. Shaker HS, Hassouna M. Sacral nerve root neuromodulation: an effective treatment for refractory urge incontinence. J Urol 1998;159:1516–19.

Chapter 19

Objective evaluation of lower urinary tract symptoms: tools for the trade

Gamal Ghoniem and Usama Khater

Quality of life questionnaires

Symptoms of pelvic floor disorders are assessed in several ways starting with history, questionnaires and voiding diaries. Clinical history usually does not adequately assess the impact of the symptom on the patient's life. Questionnaires are used to record the presence and severity of pelvic floor disorders as well as their impact on the patient's activities and quality of life. They are used as tools to objectively measure a subjective phenomenon.

There are two groups of questionnaires, generic and condition-specific questionnaires. Generic questionnaires, such as the Nottingham Health Profile and Short Form 36[1] are designed to measure function and well-being in a broad range of populations and are not specific to a particular disease, treatment or age group. However, they lack sensitivity if they are used in the evaluation of specific conditions like pelvic floor disorders or urinary incontinence, as most of these patients are in good general condition. Moreover, the same situation will be seen if the generic questionnaires are used in the evaluation of the outcome of treatment or intervention. Very little change or improvement will be seen in quality of life after treatment.

Condition-specific questionnaires are designed for a particular disease and focus on clinically important areas for the disease. Disease-specific measures or questionnaires offer greater sensitivity for the evaluation of a specific condition and are more applicable for clinical use.

There are common features of generic and condition-specific questionnaires; both of which contain a variable number of domains that gather information focused on particular aspects of health and quality of life.

Purposes of questionnaires

1. To establish the symptom or complaint.
2. To assess the severity of the symptom.
3. To measure the impact of urinary incontinence on quality of life.
4. To evaluate the treatment outcome in research and clinical settings.

Qualities of a good questionnaire

1. **Validity:** The validity of the questionnaire is whether it measures what is intended. There are three major aspects of validity.

    (a) Content: The questionnaire should make sense to those being measured, to experts in the clinical area, and the important and relevant domains should be included. The questions should be understandable to the patients and clinically sensible.
    (b) Construct validity: Examination of the ability of the questionnaire to differentiate between patient groups with different diagnoses.
    (c) Criterion validity: The level at which the questionnaire correlates with the gold standard measure that already exists.

2. **Reliable:** Reliability means the ability of the questionnaire to measure in a reproducible fashion. Reliability involves two aspects:

    (a) Internal consistency, which is the extent to which items within the questionnaire are related to each other and is measured by Cronbach's coefficient alpha.
    (b) Reproducibility is the assessment of the variability between and within observers. The questionnaire should be able to measure the same issue or symptoms in the same person over a period of time; otherwise it cannot be used in pre- and post-treatment evaluation. Stability is assessed by a test–retest analysis, where the questionnaire is given to the same set of respondents twice usually within an interval of 2–6 weeks.

3. **Responsive:** the ability to measure change of varying levels including treatment effects for different groups.

Methods of scoring

1. Simple additive: Some questionnaires may be constructed as profiles. Profiles contain a number of domains, each of which has its own score.
2. Multiplicatory scores: Scores from one type of questionnaire multiplied by scores from another and then added together to reach a total score.
3. Weighted scores: When this scoring method is used, the questionnaire includes certain symptoms, which are more significant or severe than others. High scores are assigned to the items related to these symptoms.
4. No score assigned: The questionnaires are descriptive and without scores. They are used to assess the prevalence of particular symptoms.

International implementation

For the questionnaire to be used by different cultures, several steps are suggested:

- Translation of the questionnaire.
- Back translation into the original language.
- Committee review of translations.
- Pretesting for equivalence using bilinguals.

Application of questionnaires

Quality of life questionnaires have become a recognized way to assess the impact of symptoms on patients' lives, as reporting only the symptoms in the clinical history usually offers little insight into their impact on the patient's life. Quality of life is a concept encompassing an individual's perceived level of physical, psychosocial and social well-being. The term is influenced by a broad spectrum of human experiences including diseases, accidents, treatments, interpersonal relationships and social support. A patient's quality of life is equally important as his physical status or disease, as the World Health Organization defined health as not merely absence of disease, but complete physical, mental and social well-being.[2]

Questionnaires may be long and detailed for use in research, but need to be short and easy to use to be relevant to clinical practice. In addition to being valid and reliable, they need to be easy to complete, and if they are being used to measure outcome, sensitive to change.

Frequently used questionnaires in pelvic floor disorders

UDI and IIQ questionnaires

Two popular measures developed in the United States, the Urogenital Distress Inventory (UDI) and the Incontinence Impact Questionnaire (IIQ), focus on the inconvenience of a woman's symptoms.[3] Both questionnaires are often used together, and they were specifically designed for females with urinary incontinence. They have been extensively tested in this population and shown to be valid and reliable.

The UDI consists of 19 questions relating to symptoms. Each question format is "Do you experience symptom X?" The answer is yes or no, and if yes how much does it bother you? When the subject does not have the symptom, she can skip to the next question. Each response is coded 1–4 and no response is treated as "not at all" and coded 1. The items of UDI are arranged in three subscales: irritative symptoms (6 items), obstructive/

discomfort (11 items) and stress symptoms (2 items). A mean is calculated over all questions in a subscale, and a calculation is performed so the value ranges from 0 to 100. The three subscales are summed, giving a total score of between 0 and 300. Higher scores indicate more inconvenience of symptoms.

The IIQ consists of 30 questions about the effect of urinary incontinence on the patient's quality of life (i.e., "Has urine leakage affected your ability to do Y?") and scored in a similar way to UDI.

The IIQ consists of four subscales: (1) physical activity: 6 items; (2) travel: 6 items; (3) social relationships: 10 items; and (4) emotional health: 8 items. The mean of responses is transformed to a score ranging from 0 to 100. A total score from 0 to 400 is calculated, combining the four subscores. A high score indicates greater impact of urinary incontinence.

Short forms of IIQ and UDI

Multiple regression analyses suggested that 7–8 items from the IIQ questionnaire would also accurately predict the IIQ long form total score. One item of "social activities" predicted the social/relationships subscale well. Choosing this item and the best two items of the other three IIQ subscales provided a 7–item short form (Figure 19.1).[4]

In the short form of the UDI questionnaire, Ubersax et al. found after choosing two items from each subscale, the 6–item form would accurately predict the long form total score. The resulting 6–item short form is termed the UDI-6 (Figure 19.2).

Scoring for IIQ-7

Item responses are assigned values of 0 for "not at all", 1 for "slightly", 2 for "moderately", and 3 for "greatly". For missing responses, the average score of items responded, rather than the total, is taken. The average is multiplied by 33.3 to put scores on a scale of 0 to 100. Omission of a single item from the short form will not affect the validity of the total score, however, a slight decrement in the validity will occur with omission of two items.

Bristol Female Lower Urinary Tract Symptoms (BFLUTS)

This questionnaire was developed in the UK for use with women.[5] The questionnaire covers all symptoms pertaining to female lower urinary tract symptoms. It is used for measuring changes following intervention and is a useful tool for comparing the efficacy of different treatments.

INCONTINENCE IMPACT QUESTIONNAIRE

INSTRUCTIONS

You have certain activities you do in carrying on your life. We are interested in learning what effect, if any, urinary incontinence and/or prolapse has had on these activities. The questions below refer to ways in which your activities might have changed. For each question, mark (X) the response that indicates to what extent activities have been affected by urine leakage and/or prolapse.

MR#: | 0 | 0 | 0 | 0 | 0 | | | | | | |

Patient name: _____

Has urine leakage and/or prolapse affected your:					
1. Ability to physically do the following household chores: cooking, cleaning, laundry?	☐ not at all	☐ rarely	☐ frequently	☐ all of the time	☐ not applicable
2. Ability to participate in physical recreation: walking, swimming, other?	☐ not at all	☐ rarely	☐ frequently	☐ all of the time	☐ not applicable
3. Ability to travel to entertainment activities: movies, concerts, etc?	☐ not at all	☐ rarely	☐ frequently	☐ all of the time	☐ not applicable
4. Ability to travel by car or bus more than 30 minutes from home?	☐ not at all	☐ rarely	☐ frequently	☐ all of the time	☐ not applicable
5. Participation in social/relationship activities outside of the home?	☐ not at all	☐ rarely	☐ frequently	☐ all of the time	☐ not applicable
6. Emotional health?	☐ not at all	☐ rarely	☐ frequently	☐ all of the time	☐ not applicable
7. Feeling frustrated?	☐ not at all	☐ rarely	☐ frequently	☐ all of the time	☐ not applicable

CONFIDENTIAL

Figure 19.1 Incontinence Impact Questionnaire (IIQ)-7.

King's Health Questionnaire

The King's Health Questionnaire was designed primarily for an English-speaking population. It has been used in the evaluation of different medical treatments for overactive bladder and different surgical procedures for

UROGENITAL DISTRESS INVENTORY

INSTRUCTIONS
You may have certain symptoms that indicate the
type of urinary incontinence you are experiencing.
The questions below refer to ways in which we
may learn about your incontinence. For each
question, mark (X) the response that indicates
your symptoms.

MR#: | 0 | 0 | 0 | 0 | 0 | | | | |

Visit date: | | | | 2 | 0 |

Date of birth: | | | | 1 | 9 |

Patient name: _____

Do you experience, and, if so, how much are you bothered by:					
1. Frequent urination?	☐ not at all	☐ rarely	☐ frequently	☐ all of the time	☐ not applicable
2. Urine leakage related to the feeling of urgency?	☐ not at all	☐ rarely	☐ frequently	☐ all of the time	☐ not applicable
3. Urine leakage related to physical activity: coughing or sneezing?	☐ not at all	☐ rarely	☐ frequently	☐ all of the time	☐ not applicable
4. Small amounts (drops) of urine leakage?	☐ not at all	☐ rarely	☐ frequently	☐ all of the time	☐ not applicable
5. Difficulty emptying your bladder?	☐ not at all	☐ rarely	☐ frequently	☐ all of the time	☐ not applicable
6. Pain or discomfort in the lower abdominal or genital area?	☐ not at all	☐ rarely	☐ frequently	☐ all of the time	☐ not applicable

CONFIDENTIAL

Figure 19.2 Urogenital Distress Inventory (UDI).

SUI.[6,7] The questionnaire consists of 30 questions arranged in 8 domains, namely general health perceptions, urinary symptoms, role limitations, physical-social limitations, personal relationships, emotions, sleep-energy disturbance, and incontinence impact. The scores of each domain range between 0 and 100. The higher the score, the greater impairment on quality of life.

Urgency Perception Scale (UPS)

The symptoms of overactive bladder (OAB) include urinary urgency and frequency, with or without urge incontinence. Urgency is a central and particularly bothersome hallmark symptom of OAB because it is unpredictable and consequently affects daily living.

To assess the impact of urgency, the urgency perception scale (UPS) was developed. It had been primarily used in evaluation of the efficacy of one of the antimuscarinic drugs, tolterodine, in the treatment of OAB. The USP is a single-item, three-response question.[8] The patient is asked to describe his/her typical experience when he/she feels the desire to urinate. The response options are: (1): "I am usually not able to hold urine"; (2): "I am usually able to hold urine until I reach the toilet if I go immediately"; and (3): "I am usually able to finish what I am doing before going to toilet". For the evaluation of treatment for OAB with the UPS, the range of scores is from (-2 to $+2$). Zero is coded as unchanged, negative scores as worsened, and positive as improvement.

Overactive Bladder Questionnaire (OAB-q)

OAB-q is a disease-specific questionnaire that assesses a symptom's impact on patients with OAB. The questionnaire consists of an eight-item symptom bother scale and a 25–item HRQL scale divided into four domains: coping, concern/worry, sleep and social interaction.[9]

Interstitial Cystitis questionnaires

Interstitial cystitis (IC) is a chronically progressive debilitating syndrome that substantially impacts on the patient's quality of life; two sets of validated instruments have been described in the literature. In 1997, O'Leary et al. developed a questionnaire specifically to assess IC patients.[10] The questionnaire has two sections: symptoms and problem indices. The maximum scores for each section are 20 and 16, respectively. The IC system index demonstrated internal consistency reliability, is responsive to change, and is valuable in studies of IC treatment.

A second questionnaire, the University of Wisconsin IC Scale (UW-ICS) has been developed and validated.[11] The UW-ICS is a 7-point, 0–6 rating scale with each item anchored between the extreme of 0 (not at all) to 6 (a lot). The summated rating scale has values ranging from 0 to 42.

Bladder Condition Perception (BP)

BP is a single-item self-assessment of perceived bladder condition severity used in patients at baseline and after intervention. Patients rated their perceived bladder condition severity on a six-point rating scale: 1 = no problem; 2 = very minor problems; 3 = minor problems; 4 = moderate problems; 5 = severe problems; and 6 = many severe problems. To assess treatment benefit, the patient is asked if there was any benefit from treatment. The responses are: "No", "Yes little benefit" and "Yes much benefit".

Patient Global Impression (PGI) questionnaires

Patient global impression questionnaires are assessment tools that ask the patient to rate the severity of a specific condition or to rate the response to her or his treatment. The goal of the PGI questionnaires is to get an overall appraisal of a condition, not to evaluate every component part of that condition. There are two PGI scales used for evaluation of urinary incontinence, patient global impression of severity (PGI-S) (Figure 19.3) and patient global impression of improvement (PGI-I) (Figure 19.4).

The two global indexes PGI-S and PGI-I were validated for baseline severity and for treatment response in a population of women with stress urinary incontinence in the USA.[12]

Quality of life questionnaires in fecal incontinence

According to the severity of symptoms, fecal incontinence can be classified as major or minor. Major incontinence is involuntary loss of stool. Minor incontinence consists of the loss of control of gas or occasionally liquid stool soiling. Condition-specific questionnaires can assess the degree and frequency of incontinence and its effect on quality of life. One of these questionnaires, which is used at our institution, is the Cleveland Clinic Florida/Wexner – Fecal Incontinence Scale (CCF-FIS) (Figure 19.5). This questionnaire assesses the degree and frequency of incontinence and its effect on quality of life in a numeric assessment. Such a questionnaire or scale permits objective comparison of levels of incontinence within groups

---

Patient Global Impression of Severity (PGI-S)

Check the number that best describes how
your urinary tract condition is now:

1. Normal
2. Mild
3. Moderate
4. Severe

Figure 19.3 Patient Global Impression of Severity (PGI-S) scale.

Patient Global Impression of
Improvement (PGI-I) Scale

Check the one number that best describes how your
urinary tract condition is now, compared with how it
was before you began taking medication in this study

1.   Very much better
2.   Much better
3.   A little better
4.   No change
5.   A little worse
6.   Much worse
7.   Very much worse

Figure 19.4 Patient Global Impression of Improvement (PGI-I) scale.

	Frequency			
Incontinence Never	Rarely	Sometimes	Usually	Always
Solid 0	1	2	3	4
Liquid 0	1	2	3	4
Gas 0	1	2	3	4
Wears Pad 0	1	2	3	4
Lifestyle 0 alteration	1	2	3	4
Quantified Continence Score = 20				

Never = 0, Rarely = < 1/month, Sometimes = < 1/week, > 1/month,
Usually = < 1/day, > 1/week, always = > 1/day

Figure 19.5 Cleveland Clinic Florida – Fecal Incontinence Scale (CCF-FIS).

of patients. Moreover, it permits comparison of the preoperative and postoperative values, hence the treatment results.

The CCF-FIS is scored by adding all points of the patient's response. Zero means perfect continence and 20 is complete fecal incontinence.

Short form of Pelvic Organ Prolapse/Urinary Incontinence Sexual Questionnaire (PISQ-12)

The PISQ-12 is a validated and reliable short form questionnaire that evaluates sexual function in heterosexual women with urinary incontinence and/or pelvic organ prolapse.[13] It is a condition-specific questionnaire, and it predicts the score of the long form PISQ-31.

PISQ-12 consists of 12 questions related to sexual function, effects of urinary incontinence and prolapse on sexual activity, and two questions about the male partner (Figure 19.6). Each question has 4 responses or answers and the score of the question ranges between 0 and 4. The scores are calculated by totaling the score of each question. If there is a missed value or question, the scores are calculated by multiplying the number of items by the mean of the answered items. If there are more than two missing responses, the questionnaire no longer accurately predicts long form scores.

Predictors of quality of life impairment for women with pelvic floor disorders

It is reasonable to expect that pelvic floor disorders affect the quality of life of patients. There are several factors that influence the perception of these disorders as a significant health problem. These include age, marital status, culture, social class, and duration of symptoms. A high percentage of elderly women with genitourinary symptoms feel them to be normal for elderly people. They often present for evaluation and treatment later than at younger ages. Women with detrusor overactivity have a greater quality of life impairment than those with genuine stress urinary incontinence. Interpersonal and sexual problems appear to be particularly common among urinary incontinent women, and greater for women with detrusor overactivity than for SUI. It appears that pelvic floor disorders affect different people in different ways, and in this respect QOL assessment is particularly important.

PELVIC ORGAN PROLAPSE/ URINARY
INCONTINENCE SEXUAL FUNCTION QUESTIONNAIRE

INSTRUCTIONS

The following is a list of questions about you and your partner's sex life. All information is strictly confidential. Your answers will be used only to help doctors understand what is important to patients about their sex lives. Please check the box (X) that best answers the question for you. While answering the questions, consider your sexuality over the past **six months**.

MR#: | 0 | 0 | 0 | 0 | 0 | | | | | | |

Patient name: _____

☐ This questionnaire is Not Applicable to me

	always	usually	sometimes	seldom	never
1. How frequently do you feel sexual desire? This feeling may include wanting to have sex, planning to have sex, feeling frustrated due to lack of sex, etc.	☐	☐	☐	☐	☐
2. Do you climax (have an orgasm) when having sexual intercourse with your partner?	☐	☐	☐	☐	☐
3. Do you feel sexually excited (turned on) when having sexual activity with your partner?	☐	☐	☐	☐	☐
4. How satisfied are you with the variety of sexual activities in your current sex life?	☐	☐	☐	☐	☐
5. Do you feel pain during sexual intercourse?	☐	☐	☐	☐	☐
6. Are you incontinent of urine (leak urine) with sexual activity?	☐	☐	☐	☐	☐
7. Does fear of incontinence (either stool or urine) restrict your sexual activity?	☐	☐	☐	☐	☐
8. Do you avoid sexual intercourse because of bulging in the vagina (either the bladder, rectum, or vagina falling out)?	☐	☐	☐	☐	☐
9. When you have sex with your partner, do you have negative emotional reactions such as fear, disgust, shame, or guilt?	☐	☐	☐	☐	☐
10. Does your partner have a problem with erections that affects your sexual activity?	☐	☐	☐	☐	☐
11. Does your partner have a problem with premature ejaculation that affects your sexual activity?	☐	☐	☐	☐	☐

12. Compared to orgasms you have had in the past, how intense are the orgasms you have had in the past 6 months?

☐ much less intense ☐ less intense ☐ same intensity ☐ more intense ☐ much more intense

CONFIDENTIAL

Figure 19.6 Pelvic Organ Prolapse/Urinary Incontinence Sexual Function Questionnaire (PISQ-12).

References

1. Ware JE Jr, Sherbourne CD. The MOS 36–item short-form health survey (SF-36). Conceptual framework and item selection. Med Care 1992;30:473–83.
2. World Health Organization: Definition of health from preamble to the constitution of the WHO basic documents, edn 28 (abst.). Geneva; 1978:1.
3. Shumaker SA, Wyman JF, Ubersax JS, McClish, Fantl JA. Health-related quality of life measures for women with urinary incontinence: the Incontinence Impact Questionnaire and Urogenital Distress Inventory. Quality of Life Research 1994;3:291–306.
4. Ubersax JS, Wyman JF, Shumaker SA, McClish DK, Fantl JA and the Incontinence Program For Women Research Group. Short Forms to assess life quality and symptoms for Urinary Incontinence Impact Questionnaire and Urogenital Distress Inventory. Neurourol Urodyn 1995;141:131–9.
5. Jackson S, Donovan J, Brooks S, Eckford S, Swithinbank L, Abrams P. The Bristol Female Lower Urinary Tract Symptoms questionnaire: development and psychometric testing. Br J Urol 1996;77:805–12.
6. Bidmead J, Cardozo LD, McLellan A, Khullar V, Kelleher CJ. A comparison of the objective and subjective outcomes of colposuspension for stress urinary incontinence in women. BJOG 2001;108:408–13.
7. Kobelt G, Kirchberger I, Malone-Lee[AQ1]. Quality of life aspect of the overactive bladder and the effect of treatment with tolterodine. BJU Int 1999;8:583–90.
8. Cardozo L, Coyne KS, Verse E. Validation of the urgency perception scale. BJU Int 2005;95m(4):591–6.
9. Coyne KS, Revicki DA, Hunt TL, et al. Psychometric validation of an overactive bladder symptom and health related of life questionnaire: the OAB-q. Qual Life Res 2002;11:563–74.
10. O'Leary MP, Sant GR, Fowler FJ, et al. The interstitial cystitis symptom index and problem index. Urology 1997;49:58–63.
11. Goin JE, Olaleye D, Peters KM, et al. Psychometric analysis of the University of Wisconsin Interstitial Cystitis Scale: Implications for use for use in randomized clinical trials. J Urol 1998;159:1085–90.
12. Yalcin I, Bump RC. Validation of two global questionnaires for incontinence. Am J Obstet Gynecol. 2003;89(1):98–101.
13. Roger RG, Coats KW, Kammerer-Doak, Khalsa S, Qualls C. A short form of the Pelvic Organ Prolapse/Urinary Incontinence Sexual Questionnaire (PISQ-12). Int Urogynecol J Pelvic Floor Dysfunct 2003;14(3):164–8.

Index

Page numbers in *italics* refer to tables and figures.

T - #0035 - 101024 - C16 - 234/169/17 [19] - CB - 9781841843988 - Gloss Lamination